T0190400

Adolescent Risk Behavior and Self-Regulation

Franz Resch • Peter Parzer

Adolescent Risk Behavior and Self-Regulation

A Cybernetic Perspective

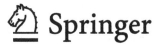 Springer

Franz Resch
Clinic for Child and Adolescent Psychiatry
University Hospital Heidelberg
Heidelberg
Germany

Peter Parzer
Clinic for Child and Adolescent Psychiatry
University Hospital Heidelberg
Heidelberg
Germany

ISBN 978-3-030-69957-4   ISBN 978-3-030-69955-0   (eBook)
https://doi.org/10.1007/978-3-030-69955-0

This Springer imprint is published by the registered company Springer Nature Switzerland AG
The registered company address is: Gewerbestrasse 11, 6330 Cham, Switzerland

Contents

Chapter 1
Adolescence

Adolescence marks the important transition from childhood to adult age. The secondary sexual characteristics make up adult appearance and habits on the basis of sexual hormones. Due to neuro-endocrine challenges various developmental processes of the brain circuits start to emerge leading to differentiations of neuronal networks by pruning processes. These changes of the brain and the adaptation requirements of teen and twen ages shape the psyche of youngsters during an "emergent adulthood".

Every adult may remember these years of conflicting emotions, dissatisfaction, distortions of the body image, desire of freedom, hopes and passions, and within feelings of fear, the attempts to live differently than the parents. The ups and downs of emotions and self-confidence have to be noticed. Bad moods and impatience raise fears of missing something important, or create concerns not to meet the requirements of the adult world. The guiding idea of a future improvement stabilizes the turmoils of mood.

Five out of six adolescents master the transition to adulthood in a satisfactory way within their social environment. However, many psychiatric disturbances of adulthood are rooted in this age period—already at the age of 14, up to 50% of psychiatric illnesses have manifested themselves in at least subclinical symptoms [1]. In Europe, around 61% of the young people are at behavioral risk, 12.5% were found to require subsequent mental health care [2]. Worldwide, 13.4% of children and adolescents seem to be affected by a psychiatric disorder [3]. Although so many youngsters (more than 80%) fulfill the developmental tasks of adolescence, the search for a new orientation within the bio-psycho-social demands of this developmental period poses a challenge for the adaptation skills of the juvenile subject.

© The Author(s), under exclusive license to Springer Nature
Switzerland AG 2021
F. Resch, P. Parzer, *Adolescent Risk Behavior and Self-Regulation*,
https://doi.org/10.1007/978-3-030-69955-0_1

1.1   Adolescence and the Brain

In the beginning basic definitions should be made. Under the term of *puberty*, the physical changes by hormonal control are summarized. These physical changes are related to body growth, sexual maturity, differentiation of sexual organs, and the appearance of secondary sexual characteristics. The maturation steps are associated with significant structural and functional changes in the brain. There are interactions between hormone production and brain development: the gonadal hormones are neuroactive substances. They influence sensory processes and the activity of the autonomic nervous system [4]. The receptor density for gonadal and adrenal (e.g. cortisol) hormones is particularly high in the brain regions, which are responsible for the transfer and interpretation of sensory information and trigger the emotional experience. These are the structures hypothalamus, amygdala, septum, and hippocampus [4].

While the physical development of puberty in girls usually begins at the age of 11, it starts in boys one and a half to 2 years later. The maturation of brain structures takes place in different regions at different times. The prefrontal cortex—which we view as the carrier of higher cognitive functions and personality performance—matures significantly later than those brain areas, that control sensory, motor, or emotional regulatory performance [5]. From a functional point of view, the anatomical reorganization of the brain allows further development of cognitive processes that control thinking, self-control, and action, allowing more flexible adaptation to the complex challenges of the natural and social environment. From a neurobiological perspective, the increased risk taking and lack of self-control of adolescents and young adults may be attributed to a differential reorganization of the adolescent brain: the hypothesis is that those subcortical areas—such as the limbic system and the reward system—develop earlier to mature than the prefrontal ones—creating an imbalance between mature subcortical and immature prefrontal structures. Intentionality and emotionality are fully developed while the control mechanisms remain immature. Imbalances between reward-driven behavior and the ability to self-regulate may be the consequence [6]. Thus, this imbalance of maturation in different brain regions could provide the cerebral substrate for increased impulsivity and risk taking in adolescents [7]. The dual systems explanatory model for adolescent risk behavior has been a dominant framework for the past decade to conceptualize the mechanisms underlying these adolescent behavior features [8].

However, brain development based on gene-driven maturation does not take place in empty space. Environmental influences have a modifying effect. Intense and extraordinary experiences, but also drug effects and nutritional factors have a specific impact on the functional organization of the brain. There is a "neuronal plasticity", which forms a structural memory of the environment. Neuronal maps of the environment are displayed in brain structures. Psychological traumas in this context have a strong influence on the functional organization and maturation processes of the brain. Childhood maltreatment is associated with continuing effects on brain development during adolescence [9].

There is evidence, that sleep duration may impact the risk-taking behavior through its effect on the brain [10]. Transient interference in the right dorsolateral prefrontal cortex has been reported to result in heightened risk taking among young adults caused by failure to inhibit risky decisions while increasing cortical excitability in this area seemed to diminish risk taking [11]. Following sleep loss, changes of prefrontal cortex functioning were similarly observed. Furthermore, adolescents who obtained less sleep had a reduced reactivity of reward related brain regions like the caudate of the ventral striatum in anticipation of a reward. As a consequence, adolescents may seek more exciting or risky rewards to experience satisfaction [10]. Life style shapes brain development by shaping brain functions.

Adolescence encompasses the maturation processes of puberty and integrates them into psychosocial developmental stages towards adulthood. It therefore covers a period of more than 10 years. It is characterized by a series of changes. Adolescence is a very culturally sensitive phase.

1.2 Adolescence and Emergent Adulthood

Brain development is associated with functional development of the cognitive and emotional areas, including an increase in working memory and information processing speed. Thinking reaches the abstract levels of problem definition and stepwise problem solution.

There is an increase in knowledge and skills in various domains of reality, especially in the field of social cognition. The issues of emotional regulation and self-control will be addressed later in Chap. 3.

In an increasingly complex globalizing world, young people face challenges that affect both the public and private sphere. In most Western countries, for example, young people should attain the highest possible level of education in order to have the best possible chances in the increasingly competitive labor market. Young people who fail because of mental problems in the education and training sector, thus come under additional pressure: they endanger their professional and personal future through their mental crisis [12].

In addition, everyday life is so strongly influenced by the new media that children are really surrounded by music streams, videos, television, smartphones, computers, and various ways of internet offers [13]. On the one hand, young people are given a very open access to information, they are given communicative spaces and creative opportunities; on the other hand, it may be difficult to find the right choice in this abundance of offers. It is difficult, not to be distracted by fake news, not getting bogged down in games and self-presentations on the internet [12]. While the adult generation can contribute their own experiences to the use of media such as television, radio, magazines, or books, the new media such as computers, the internet and mobile phones have created a potential for use that shapes young people's growth in a specifically different way with its interactive structures compared to the parent generation [13]. After all, the new media have become an integral part of the everyday life of adolescents, and the increased interactivity makes it fundamentally possible to reorganize social action in the net [13]. Although the importance of virtual social networks and the long-term presence of mobile phones for the mental development process have not yet been fully recognized, we must certainly say goodbye to older theories of the development of personality before the new media or revise these theories, which are based primarily on direct interpersonal contact. Peer relations may also be transformed in the social media context providing new opportunities of friendship and relational maintenance behavior. However evidence has begun to accumulate that reassurance- and feedback-seeking behaviors do occur on social media and may exert negative consequences for youth leading to the adoption of risky behaviors [14].

Media have an impact on developmental tasks such as identity development, autonomy demands, and separation from the home. As adolescents are often superior to their parents in dealing with the so-called new media, they are able to move around in virtual environments, encounter unknowns, get to know opportunities and risky practices, try out new relationships, and start a new form of replacement of the parents in close proximity to them [13].

We conclude: With these new media, a great potential for personal development has emerged that, with its interactive structures, shapes the life of adolescents in a completely different way than the parent generation knows from their own youth. New forms of interactive problems also manifest themselves in the form of cyberbullying and suicide forums, in which adolescents can be negatively influenced. What impact this will have on the development of personalities in the future, we cannot even say today. However, it is clear that the simple rejection, or prohibition, of social media tends to inhibit, rather than encourage, young people in their development! Anyone who warns about "digital dementia" [15] overlooks the fact that emancipation is only possible today through the inclusion of the media worlds [16]!

Developmental psychologists, such as Arnett [17] and Seiffge-Krenke [18], therefore, propose the term "emerging adulthood", that defines a prolonged adolescence characterized by the temporal extension and complication of the transition from adolescent lifestyle to a responsible adult position [19]. New forms of intergenerational coexistence, the broadening of the spectrum of social roles, and the increasing complexity of educational pathways in a world of new information technologies are blamed for this [18]. While Arnett [17] still spoke of "fun and exploration", Seiffge-Krenke [18] makes it clear that the ruminative search for one's own social role and impact can also be very painful and involves mental problems.

1.3   Development and Developmental Tasks

Development means differentiation. The developmental concept that underlies the considerations on "risk behavior and cybernetics" is based on an interactionist model of development [20]. This model connects an active, self-motivated subject with an equally active and influential environment. Physical conditions, cultural techniques, rituals, objects, and attachment figures serve as developmental incentives or challenges, that the individual has to deal with [21]. The individual is ascribed an equally active role in shaping the environment as the individual is affected and shaped by the latter [22].

The concept of developmental tasks by Havighurst [23] shares with other developmental concepts—like Anna Freud's [24] developmental lines—the ideas of normative development, continuity, and sequencing. Unique, however, is the emphasis on the individual's active performance in development. By solving age-specific development tasks, one's own development can be driven forward and advanced. The focus is on individual activity. Coping with the need for adjustment becomes apparent in different forms, namely on the one hand in a successful further development or on the other hand in a development standstill or regression. To solve age-specific development tasks, requirements from three areas (physical condition, social norms, and individual abilities) must be integrated. Havighurst's approach is based on an outline of the human biography in six sections:

- Early Childhood from birth to 5–6 years.
- Middle Childhood from 5–6 years to 12–13 years.
- Adolescence from 12–13 years to 18 years.
- Early Adulthood from 18 to 35 years.
- Middle Adulthood from 35 to 60 years.
- Late Maturity 60 years and older.

For each of these six stages of development, he has defined several age-specific development tasks that are networked across the lifecycle. The developmental tasks of adolescence comprise at least:

- The re-conceptualization of the self,
- the development of a mature body concept,
- the replacement of the parents,
- the development of mature relationships with close friends, and
- the beginning of romantic relationships.

These are based on the successful developmental tasks of late childhood (e.g. learning physical skills, building a positive attitude towards oneself as a growing organism, learning an appropriate gender (or transgender) role, achieving personal independence).

The realization of coping with the development tasks in turn represents the prerequisite for the initiation of the phase-specific development tasks of the next age group.

In Havighurst's conception, the normative claim of society on development is emphasized much more clearly than in other developmental concepts: Many developmental tasks include normative expectations such as school entry, transition to a secondary school, graduation, etc. The sequencing of developmental tasks is also explicitly operationalized. Developmental tasks, especially in childhood and adolescence, have been well studied [25]. Developmental tasks are also subject to the Zeitgeist and may change with the historical development. They are not simply

determined by nature but are socially designed. Developmental tasks can be culturally different and form different emphases in different cultures. New definitions of
developmental tasks in the context of new media still need to be done.

1.4   The Problem of Identity

Who am I—is the central question of man. It is an expression of self-awareness.
With the age of puberty and adolescence, the child enters a developmental phase of
extended self-reflective possibilities. Does your own mentalization reflect reality?
Does it depict a reality that also exists outside the cognitive process, or is your own
world experience only illusory, an inner construct, an illusion that also disappears
with the disappearance of the thinker? These philosophical problems not only
occupy the academic institutions for centuries but every young person who is seeking to approach the outside world and its own self.

Identity characterizes the correspondence between the subject and himself. The
living person experiences his or her actions through a self-reflective process as a
unit. Identity is thus an act of self-positioning of the individual in different perspectives: the immediate experience of experiencing oneself in one's own actions is
reconciled with the self-observations. Historically, we assume that the concept of
identity—as we understand it today—has much to do with the advent of the
European Enlightenment. The Enlightenment, which connects the specific human
being with "the reason", has to struggle with the problem that we find in each human
emotional abysses, which can be brought under the sphere of influence of the rational only with the greatest effort, so the reason-human must live in constant concern
of impending self-loss [26].

The unity of the person is more difficult to achieve than the Enlightenment might
have promised us. We are not slotted together by an inner relationship of domina-
tion, we are not a unity by authority, but must achieve a balance between different
polarities through an inner dialectic [19].

The identity of man comes from two main sources [27]. The first source is the
reflective experience of identity: Identity is a self-perception as unique and unmistakable from the outside, as well as an inward agreement between first- and third-
person perspectives. The ego as a self-conscious actor is matched with the self as an
object of self-consideration. The manifold flows of the person become an indivisible
and unmistakable whole. The reflective identity has been described in its components by Scharfetter [28] from a psychopathological point of view. In the field of
infant research, these dimensions could be confirmed from a developmental psychology perspective [29, 30]. The reflective identity is based on basic experiences
of one's own "vitality" (the sense of being alive) and one's own "activity"—whereby
the reference copy of one's own actions is the basis of self-reliance [31]. The "consistency" is a feeling of inner homogeneity across different emotional states and the
"coherence", a basic feeling of the continuity of selfhood over different stages of
development. Finally, the reflective identity is characterized by a fundamental

experience of "demarcation" from within and without, from self and others. If the demarcation is lost, the fear of a dangerous merger arises.

In addition to this reflective experience of identity, there is a second mechanism of identity construction—identification. The identification of subjects with persons or individual characteristics of persons, with idols or ideals, is assigned to their own self and benefits it. We can also identify with (social) roles and tasks that then appear as self-determining goals of the person. An important aspect of identification is the concept of belonging to defined groups or political parties, religious communities, or ethnic groups, which define our participation through recognition and acceptance. Belonging to a confirming community strengthens the sense of identity. Being recognized by the other members of the community plays a fundamental role in this respect [27].

In adolescents, identification processes can become effective not only through affiliations and social roles but also through their own creative activity—forming objects—for which a concept of "expressive identity" [32] stands. Through a creative process, objects can be produced, with which one can identify oneself, objects that can establish relationships with others and can be presented to other people as a substitute for the self. In this way, adolescents in social roles can express their own abilities, talents, and interests through activities in pieces of work (paintings, poems, performances, technical objects)—while gaining self-security from interaction with others by applying the process of identification [12].

There is a dialectic relationship between the reflective identity and the identification identity, and this opposition between demarcation and participation reveals an essential basic problem of the concept of identity: A reflective experience of identity defined by self-centeredness and differentiation from others is confronted with an identification identity that is centered around belonging, community, and opening up to others who recognize one [12]. In such groups, who define themselves strongly by belonging, however, there is an irrefutable tendency to differentiate from others outside the group, which in turn means an exclusion of "foreigners" in addition to—and as a dark side of—the experience of belonging. In this search for validation in groups, there may be a risk of temptation and seduction when the needy individual joins radical, political, or religious groups in his search for belonging. Adolescents may be seduced into aggression, drug use, or criminal activities just to be part of it. On the other hand, self-reflective identity, if it succeeds in maintaining internal diversity and creates a polyvalent self, becomes an important element of tolerance [19].

Looking at the ontogenetic history of human development from infancy to adulthood, both processes of identity formation are based on a fundamental, interactive environmental resonance. After all, the mentalization process, the ability to reflect environmental conditions, the "inner world" of the adolescents, are rooted together in the child's dialogue with his important caregivers [33]. The development of cognitions and reflections takes a route from the outside world of interaction to an inner mental space in which self-reflection is possible [21, 34].

Since the development of identity begins in childhood and continues as an emotional dialogue into adulthood [27]—i.e. the development of identity remains a lifelong process—in changing environments, developmental opportunities will depend crucially on these environmental conditions. The development of identity does not seem to us as a process that follows genetically from the human blueprint but requires a precarious redefinition due to the environmental situation.

Identity as a whole can always only be a momentary, emotional integration of different aspects of identity, which is internally available to the person under the goal of acting. "I can act as one even though I consist of many". We can only intellectually capture parts of ourselves. So, when we act, we live in an "illusion of unity", an emotionally mediated idea that makes us capable of action [19]. Identity must always be actively re-established. It is not an enduring insight that can be simply remembered and remains effective thereby.

Secured, loved, and recognized in their parental relationships, adolescents develop a good inner reflectivity, a stable set of self-knowledge beyond adulthood, which allows for and tolerates diversity and uncertainties in self-affirmation. These adolescents, with secure attachment and a "good enough" emotional dialogue with caregivers, have a strong and secure polyvalent sense of self based on a stable emotional regulation. These young people experience themselves as individuals in different social roles, including failures or non-recognition. They have achieved an inner emotional stability that enables a stable process of self-reflection of identity [12].

However, when adolescents have to cope with an interrupted emotional dialogue with important caregivers, when they are traumatized—e.g. having been subjected to sexual abuse or violence, having been rejected, devalued, disrespected, and humiliated, or if they have had unpredictable mentally ill parents whose desires were unbearable—then the secure inner mental space does not develop [27]. Self-reflection, identity, and self-worth remain precarious. Such adolescents are highly dependent on the identity foundation through affiliation and group belonging. They need recognition and affirmation, they become tempted against group targets such as violence or fanaticism, and they risk becoming involved. Education, attachment, and emotional dialogue are thus the social keys for mature, democracy-capable youth, in contrast to fanatical followers and subordinates [35].

The question of social identity was taken up with great sensitivity by Erikson in his development draft "Identity and the life cycle" [36]. The young people not only have to develop a sense of who they are, but also what they will be like in the future. This includes the development of personal goals, values, and the will to take responsibility. Based on Erikson's ideas, several research groups are now working on an empirical examination of identity concepts from a developmental psychological point of view (overview by [18]). There is a Canadian working group [37], a Belgian [38], and a Norwegian [39] researching the identity concept. In Germany, the working group of Seiffge-Krenke [40] equally deals with empirical research on identity, in Switzerland, it is the working group around Klaus Schmeck [41].

The model of identity is divided into two dimensions according to the approaches of Marcia [37] and the assumption is made that identity results from the probation in social roles—in the three domains "work, personal relationships, and values". The two dimensions are *exploration* and *commitment*. Exploration is the search for, the investigation, and testing of different social roles in different areas of life, while commitment involves social responsibility. It is about social roles that correspond to career, subsistence, mate choice, romantic relationships, partnership, and general aspects of meaning and value, that is, ethical awareness. The exploration of such social roles finally follows, under normal conditions, the commitment. Marcia [37] was the first to make empirical studies on identity in the 1990s.

Marcia described four different identity constellations. Normally the so-called "achieved identity" is to be expected, after sufficient exploration a binding role commitment becomes tangible. The so-called "foreclosure" finally takes place without sufficient search for alternatives through an overly early decision to take on the role. A third phenomenon is the "moratorium", where, in repeated cycles of exploration, the individual can not commit himself sufficiently to a particular social role typing. Repeated exploration attempts without liability are also referred to in the literature as ruminative exploration [18]. The fourth group is characterized by so-called "identity diffusion", which has neither an explorative search for alternatives nor a binding role commitment.

Recent work by the Norwegian working group [39] showed that only about one-third of 20-year-old adolescents in the transition to young adulthood had achieved normal identity. On the other hand, about a quarter had been found in the moratorium, that is, in the ruminative search for social possibilities. Around 20% showed identity diffusion. Marcia found in his research that since the 70s to the end of the century, an increase in diffuse identity was recorded. Similar results were also described in meta-analyzes by other authors (review by [18]). Today we assume that identity diffusion and moratorium are increasing and that the social challenges obviously require more of a social diversity than a deepening of few social roles [42].

The philosopher Descombes [32] and the social philosopher Hartmut Rosa [43] advocate the multiplicity of identities. They note that modern individualization can obviously help to escape rigidly predetermined social roles. This may liberate adolescents internally and broaden their life horizons. What is needed, however, is to maintain a balance between continuity and coherence on the one hand and changes, diversity, and flexibility on the other.

But the question arises: when does the pluralization and multiplication of the subjective self come to an end, when do fragmentation and confusion begin, when does diversity turn into chaos, when do the possibilities and chances become arbitrary, when does the great choice become a torment? At that point, in the multiplicity of opportunities, the structures of the self start to corrode, the subject begins to dissolve, as Richard Sennet [44] has described. It turns out that those individuals who have a stable identity development also endure more diversity. Those who can rely on secure emotional dialogues are more likely to sustain role diversity [19].

In contrast, in the moratorium of repetitive role-seeking or identity diffusion, young people are more prone to depression, anxiety, psychosomatic complaints, or risk behaviors [18, 42]. Combining this with the empirical fact that we have seen an increase in mental disorders over the last few decades (see Chap. 10), there seems to be a secular trend of increasing emotional problems and risk behaviors in children and adolescents, which is particularly evident in highly developed industrialized countries [45], it must be thought-provoking. We can assume that emotional problems of adolescents have increased in several European countries over the last 30 years. Risk behaviors also show this trend: are the pluralization of the self and the increase of emotional problems and risk behaviors in adolescents interrelated [19]? This question will be addressed in Chap. 10.

1.5   The Problem of Self-Worth

Narcissistic regulation—as an evaluative stabilization of self-esteem—is characterized by an in-depth assessment of one's own ability to adapt to the physical and social environment. Self-worth and the ability to act must be defended against hostility by others or failed adaptation tasks. The narcissistic regulatory system is part of a broader system of self-assurance. Self-esteem undergoes restructuring in adolescence through the intensification of self-reflective activities. However, preliminary stages of self-esteem and self-control have already taken place in earlier phases of life.

Narcissism as auto-regulatory activity includes not only the areas of self-assurance—as trust in one's own competence and trust in acceptance by others—but as well an emotional and intentional self-occupation, which in its positive form means self-acceptance and self-care. Only in a pathologically exaggerated form does narcissism appear as self-obsession, self-centeredness, and parasitism. The considerate and fearless self-centeredness without self-doubt is rare in childhood and adolescence and impresses more as cold and dullness than self-love. It usually results from the most severe early interactional disappointments and trauma [46].

Self-esteem can be briefly defined as a reflective realization of the competence and acceptance experiences that an individual makes in his engagement with the environment. We can see that components of competence and acceptance have significance for both self-esteem and identity development. How do self-esteem and identity develop? Both self-regulation and identity construction are based on the evolving competences of perspective-taking [46]. To experience the phenomenon of acceptance (someone takes me seriously), the individual must be able to empathize with others and show the competences of perspective-taking. On the other hand, self-reflective abilities are needed, to realize one's own competence and performance (the actual implementation of competences on current occasions). The toddler benefits from early forms of acceptance as attachment security: the parents are shelters and creators of the child's experiential space.

In the case of the schoolchild, self-esteem regulation succeeds through experiences of acceptance and competence—through experiences of success and through the feedback from the important caregivers. Self-esteem regulation, however, is depending on the early childhood self-structure and succeeds due to the integration of the self, up to this stage of development.

It has to be emphasized that the child's ability to integrate its self-parts should not be judged solely from an adult perspective and thus devalued. Children are optimally adapted to their individual needs at every phase of their lives and disorders of self-integration in children must always be compared to the level of integration of childhood normality [47]. In adolescence, self-regulation is complicated by the fact that peer group acceptance becomes much more important than at the school-age stage. Non-acceptance by the peer group can no longer be compensated by parental confirmation alone [12].

In the development concept of Erikson [48] the formation of self-worth and the formation of identity are seen as successively appearing developing tasks of latency and adolescence. However, this view must be contradicted. A self-esteem regulation that succeeds in school age or in the latency phase is also put to the test again in adolescence. Self-esteem and identity are not independent of each other or represent self-functions that build on each other but are interwoven processes which, in each phase of development, have to orient themselves according to new goals and establish new equilibrium [27]. Even if latency self-regulation is successful in avoiding feelings of inferiority, this regulation is no guarantee for the next phase of development. If feelings of inferiority are prevented by the subject bending his basic experiences in the interaction through self-denial or defending himself in sham adjustments and self-alienation, then despite self-confirmation's temporary success in competence and acceptance, the next step of identity development may be compromised, and subsequently self-esteem regulation may experience danger.

Self-esteem in adolescence must be constituted on a new reflective level in interaction with identity development. Noteworthy, self-esteem can never be firmly anchored to one pole of competence or the other pole of acceptance. Self-esteem is never alone competence or acceptance alone, but always both. Structurally, it should be noted that there can never be identity problems without self-esteem problems. The threatened self by disintegration or identity diffusion is always threatened in its self-esteem regulation.

Those who are not valued and encouraged by others, who are not viewed by others as attractive, whose looks and abilities cannot contribute to an improvement in self-esteem, even if they are objectively positive, are at increased risk for impending self-loss. The increased need for self-reflection and social echo can only be satisfied through successful interactions with peers and the concomitant positive social acceptance. Self-worth and identity refer to each other and depend on each other in their development [19].

Problems of identity and self-worth always play into the symptoms of mental disorders in adolescents and shape the clinical picture.

Chapter 2
Risk Behavior

2.1 Introduction and Definition

Taking risks, looking for challenges, and trying oneself out are normal adolescent needs. Every young person wants to test their limits and explore their chances. But more and more in a process of rumination these needs may become passions, may become necessary for oneself and the playful character of the risk search turns into bitter seriousness of self-definition at risk.

Not all young people master their developmental tasks satisfactorily; they get into crises of adjustment. If developmental tasks are mastered only in a difficult way, acute disturbances of adaptation may occur, which are usually accompanied and shaped by identity diffusion, self-alienation experiences, role confusion, shakes of self-esteem, as well as family-life conflicts [27]. Detachment from the primary family is complicated by such relationship issues. In adolescence adjustment problems and crises of adaptation are usually associated with risk behaviors: These are defined by patterns of behavior that mean a willful endangerment of the person, with the goals of a short-term satisfaction of needs, a momentary solution of adjustment problems, self-assurance, or simply the achievement of being recognized by peers. To increase identity and self-worth, a threat to the person and their future is accepted. Risk behaviors are thus characterized by a lack of self-care, a lack of health awareness, and a lack of social prudence, but they are basically at the service of the self! Although risk behaviors may be related to poor impulse control and decision-making, they are often used in lieu of self-regulation strategies like affect control or tolerance of negative emotions. Alcohol consumption, drug use, or self-injury may make fundamental sense to the individual, in some way, but may cause damage in the long run. If you want someone to stop this behavior, you need to offer other relief mechanisms: help them solve a problem, change their life circumstances, or gain insight. The adolescent will continue his risk behavior as long as he does not have alternative forms of self-regulation. Risk behavior is not an illness,

F. Resch, P. Parzer, *Adolescent Risk Behavior and Self-Regulation*,
https://doi.org/10.1007/978-3-030-69955-0_2

but serves a fundamental functional role [49]. Risk behavior must be replaced with more adaptive regulatory options, which is nurtured within the context of a "holding environment" [50].

Risk behaviors can be characterized by the following behavioral features in detail (modified according to [51]):

- Internet addiction,
- smoking, tobacco use and substance abuse (alcohol and drugs),
- non-suicidal self-injury (NSSI) and suicidal behavior,
- disordered eating and diets,
- adolescent aggression, violence, and delinquent behavior,
- adolescent pregnancy and sexually transmitted diseases,
- bullying and school absenteeism.

Risk behaviors are usually interrelated. They are likely to cluster, further exacerbating the social and health-related threats [2, 51]. Excessive use of alcohol and drugs may lead to addiction or to social violations, including delinquent behaviors such as theft, fraud, blackmail, or robbery. Risk behaviors can also be associated with a decrease in performance motivation, which gives rise to serious schooling and training problems. School refusal and school absenteeism currently form important adaptation problems of adolescence [52, 53]. Relationship patterns may be characterized by conflict and aggressiveness, which leads to conflicts with authorities and peer rivals. Serious quarrels may start within families—which in turn complicate the processes of juvenile detachment and emancipation from the parents [54]. Risk behaviors may also involve the new media, with addictive internet consumption often associated with encapsulation, withdrawal from social contacts, and a weakening of reality control [55]. As the sleep-wake cycle changes or dietary habits change, ascetic rituals and day-night reversals can occur. Excessive or neglected personal hygiene becomes a caricature of the necessary cultural techniques of adulthood. In extreme cases, subway surfing or power pole climbing can lead to mutual incitement in youth groups. Risky sexual behaviors are characterized by the facts that the predisposed adolescents are sexually indiscriminate, avoiding precautions with an increased risk of sexually transmitted diseases [56].

Many risk behaviors follow the pattern of "Russian Roulette": Consciously it is accepted that something bad—in the worst-case life-threatening—can happen. Not infrequently, teenagers are under the illusion of how much they can handle the dangers—which adults have found difficult to control. Such proximal thinking, which focuses only on the near future and on potential benefits, neglects the aftereffects or collateral dangers like health compromising consequences, social conflicts, or sanctions initiated by the adult world. Asceticism, curiosity and the joy of experimentation are lived out on purpose, however, they hamper the taking of responsibility in reality [56].

Risk behaviors in adolescents fulfill an individual, specific function in the course of development tasks, which can only be decrypted by a functional context analysis [57]. It appears that the emergence of risk behaviors says a lot about adolescents' current social skills. These actual adaptation capacities turn out as key factors for the occurrence of risk behaviors. Adolescents who have been impaired by a lack of social feedback, bullying experiences, or failures in school and work environments are more likely to display risk behaviors such as self-injury [58]. For adolescents seeking outreach or cliques, the strong social echo from deviant groups can lead to ever-riskier behaviors that are akin to an upswing process. Especially when parents do not seem to be available and the protective role of parental care and control is missing, the values of peers play an even bigger role, if these are meeting the youngster's needs for affirmation [56]. Thus, the dangers of risk behaviors may be particularly underestimated by youth as they are banned by or cause rejection and dismay in adults [57]. Risk behaviors lead to young people feeling better themselves; they may allow them to build a better self-image or to gain feelings of confirmation. Appreciation in these cases results precisely from the demarcation of the adult world [56]. The more adults reject and condemn these behaviors, the more likely the adolescents feel confirmed.

Risk behaviors are not equally distributed between the two sexes. While drug use and aggressive behavior seem more common among male adolescents, eating disorders and emotional regulation disorders as well as self-harm are more common in girls. Risk behaviors apparently enable adolescents to reach their proximal personal goals and thus satisfy a need for self-stabilization and recognition. In the long run, however, they create more problems than they can solve. Risk behaviors can inhibit social and educational development, endangering immediate health, causing disfiguring injuries, or alienating the family and friendly environment so that important contacts can no longer be sustained [12].

Some authors call these risk behaviors "social morbidities" to indicate, that adolescent morbidity and mortality are often the result of life-style practices among adolescents and risk behaviors represent potentially preventable causes of life threat [51]. "Lifestyle psychiatry" has recently focused on that [59].

Risk behaviors do not show a clear border to psychopathological symptoms. While risk behaviors serve more to test limits and to expand the subjective scope, psychopathological symptoms present with the character of personal suffering. They serve to compensate for grief and pain or to ward off traumatic experiences. Symptoms and risk behaviors can combine and mix and both be dedicated to the survival of the self.

2.2 Explanatory Models of Risk-Taking Behaviors

The classical framework for explaining adolescent risk behavior has been addressed in Chap. 1. The so-called dual systems model [6] states, that the incentive processing system matures earlier than the cognitive control system. Imbalances between reward-driven behavior and the ability to self-regulate may be the consequences [7]. However, recent studies have suggested, that adolescent risk behavior may be subtyped in reasoned and reactive risk behaviors [60]. Reasoned risk behavior is premeditated, with adolescents choosing purposefully to engage in activities to gain some benefit or relief, although these activities may be known to be risky. It reflects some kind of exploratory behavior. Reactive risk behavior is more impulsive, driven by a deficit in response inhibition. While reactive risk behavior may be explained well by lower executive capability, reasoned risk behavior seems to result from engagement in purposeful behavior and may be based on more mature executive functioning. A new study on 1266 participants with a mean age of 16.5 years showed, that reasoned risk behavior was associated with higher levels of sensation seeking, better working memory, greater future orientation and perceiving risk behavior more beneficial than risky—in comparison with reactive risk behaviors [8]. Thus, the prevailing framework may be challenged—adolescent risk behavior may not be explained solely by poor response inhibition! More complex models are needed including motivational and intentional aspects of behavior.

The classical bio-psycho-social models for the explanation of risk behaviors try to describe complex relationships in different domains. Many individual studies with particular relationships between somatic or social factors and the psyche are based on these models. The bio-psycho-social models always tried to relate data on different levels of abstraction in relationships of covariance. The more general these interaction models are formulated, the more comprehensively they seem to be valid, but the less their explanatory value for the individual case becomes [61]. The question is to clarify how the different perspectives of the biological, social, and psychological domains can be brought together and integrated (see Chap. 5). Data of different domains should not only correlate but also make sense in terms of content. Can the bio-psycho-social model actually produce a whole, or do the particular findings remain isolated on their levels of puzzle pieces [62]?

Can we categorize knowledge in the bio-psycho-social model in such a way that a meaningful whole results from it? If the bio-psycho-social model is intended as an integrative construct of understanding and allows each individual data set on risk behavior to be assigned a place in different domains, there is a rapidly growing desire for a uniform explanation of the whole, in which all details are defined by one theory in a regular and deterministic way [63]. At these interfaces where different fields of knowledge collide, the desire for a meta-theory or meta-language becomes urgent, which may pervade all domains of knowledge and experience and, integrating the details as it were, enables a unique bio-psycho-social formulation. However, this meta-language does not (yet) exist, even if some particular domains of science (especially the neurobiological domain) repeatedly make this general claim.

For example, neurobiological advances have vastly expanded our knowledge of brain functions, cognitive performance and the cerebral localization of mental processes [64]. Such neurobiological findings try to "substantiate" the psychic constructs as scientific phenomena. Using the medical model within a psycho-biological perspective, risk behaviors and psychological symptoms often appear as facts that can be derived from brain dysfunction and require therapy. Neurobiological findings thus may have an anti-stigmatizing effect on psychological disorders. An example of this is the construct of "dissociation", whose cerebral correlates can be clearly distinguished from processes in simulation. Dissociative paralysis is therefore something other than "pretending to be paralyzed". Even if neurobiological insights can take away the flaw of falseness and deception from mental disorders, they do not legitimize these mental disorders in the social domain. Deciphering the pathogenesis at the neurobiological level could indeed define a disease construct. But that doesn't tell us anything about the functionality of the symptoms in the individual case. The gap between categories from subjective experience to organic findings remains indissoluble (see Chap. 5).

Those who try to attribute an effect of the psychic domain on the somatic domain quickly fall into a dualistic trap. How could such effects be recorded? Influencing somatic processes by psychological processes violates the principle of the conservation of energy. Energy inputs into the physiological processes cannot emerge from mental activities. Nevertheless, psychosomatic effects are undeniable and adverse childhood events have disadvantageous effects on the psyche and soma! Symptoms (like hallucinations, depression, or aggression) are not only a result of dysfunctional somatic processes—on the contrary, they can disrupt and interrupt somatic processes by themselves. Aberrant experiences may produce aberrant cerebral processes and structures.

Are our language-systems comprehensive and differentiated enough to be able to offer the bio-psycho-social model a single meta-language for an integration of the knowledge domains? While neuroscientists see this time approaching, we as psychotherapists currently have to answer this question with a "no". A mathematically exact formulation of brain or hormonal functions may not get easily through to the description of the inner world of the subject. However, dismissing the inner world as "epi-phenomenological noise" based on closed somatic causal interpretations makes the specific domain of our therapeutic interventions disappear. Additionally, there are also no convincing translation options between the different fields of knowledge in the biological, social and psychological domains subjected to the empirical answering of questions about subjective adaptation to the environment by purposeful behavior [65]. We assume that the bio-psycho-social model cannot be formulated in the mathematical language of physics or molecular biology alone [62].

Risk behaviors cannot be sufficiently explained by a few causal pathways, which are defined by general genetic or cerebral mechanisms disregarding the individual subject and its history, but it is necessary to relate the behavior in each individual case to the developmental context and thus make it understandable. Risk behaviors are caused by multiple causes (multi-causality) and are defined in their purposes as a multi-final probability construct in the further course (multi-finality).

2.3   Risk Behavior Patterns

Risk behaviors can occur singularly in a domain (e.g. internet addiction) or present with typical combinations (e.g. NSSI and suicidal tendencies). There are different distributional patterns of combined risk behaviors that can be found empirically from population studies or cohort studies.

Studies on American adolescents were able to identify four subtypes using latent class analyzes. One group comprises "Non-sexually Active, High Risk Behavior Youth" with relatively high probabilities of engaging in delinquency—e.g. selling drugs to their peers at school, drinking and driving, or carrying a weapon. This group occurs in about 5% of the cases. Another group is labeled as "Experimenters" (36% of the cases). These youth show up with drinking and driving a car themselves, they smoke marihuana, have a high alcohol and cigarette use, and engage in gambling activities. They have multiple partners without using a condom during sexual activities. A third group may be called "High, Diverse Risk Behavior Youth", it makes up around 22% of the overall sample. Very high levels in terms of probabilities for all risk behaviors can be documented. They often get into a fight and show a high amount of delinquency, they are sexually active with multiple partners with a risk of unsafe sex. They are drug and alcohol consumers and show all sorts of risky behaviors. The fourth group makes up roughly 36% of the overall sample and is called "Abstainers". This group shows low probabilities for all risky behaviors. No sex, no drugs, no weapons. The total sample consisted of 2549 high school youth, roughly 16 years of age, sex equally distributed [66]. We can detect a rather quiet group of risk behaviors or abstainers in about 41% of the cases. However, more than 50% of the adolescents show up with behaviors that endanger their development. It is very unlikely that there is a mental illness behind all of these behaviors. After all, who wanted to believe that more than half of young people are mentally ill?

In the European SEYLE-project (Saving and Empowering Young Lives in Europe) the epidemiological data of 11,110 pupils in the age group 14 to 16 years (mean 14.8 ± 0.8) were collected [67, 68]. 10 European countries participated. Prevalence rates of various risk behaviors were obtained: alcohol use 13.4%, smoking 30.9%, physical inactivity 32.8%, pathological internet use 4.4%. The prevalence of sexual debut was 18.8% for the total sample. Three clusters of the adolescent sample could be identified [69] by a latent class analysis: A "low-risk group" (57.8%) with a low frequency of all risk behaviors, a "high-risk group" (13.2%) who scored high on all risk dimensions and an "invisible-risk group" (29%) who scored positive for high use of internet/TV/videogames, sedentary behavior and reduced sleep. Individuals of the high-risk group and the members of the invisible-risk group had similarly increased prevalence rates of anxiety, subthreshold depression, and suicidal thoughts compared to low-risk individuals. Although the studies in America and Europe cannot be compared directly due to methodological reasons, it is noticeable that the frequencies of risk behaviors seem to differ. More than 50% of the youngsters in Europe were estimated "low risk". Also, the prevalence rates of high-risk groups seem to favor European youth. But the basic problem remains: risk behaviors endanger development.

Risk behaviors rarely occur as single styles of behavior, as has been demonstrated, mostly they are correlated. There are clear connections between suicidality and self-harm, between aggressiveness, dissocial behavior, and substance abuse, or between withdrawal and risky media consumption. Changing relationships can also be found in risk behaviors with symptoms of depression, sleep disorders, and post-traumatic disorders. Risk behavior and psychopathological symptoms are interrelated, risk behavior causes, initiates or accelerates mental disorders (e.g. the relationship between smoking habits, substance abuse and addiction, or between self-harm, depression and suicidality). On the other hand, psychopathological symptoms are attempted to be compensated for with risk behavior (e.g. depressive moods are attempted to be compensated for with substance abuse, or serious self-esteem and identity disorders with aggressive self-assertion).

One factor comprising all forms of risk behaviors that may heighten the risk-taking propensity is lack of sleep. A systematic review of evidence examining the relationship between sleep duration and risk-taking in adolescents has been presented by Short and Weber [10]. Studies including 579,380 individuals were evaluated. Pooled results indicated that shorter sleep was associated with increased odds of risk-taking behavior—e.g. cigarette smoking, alcohol and drug use, sexual risk-taking or violence. However, the empirical evidence of an association between sleep and risk behavior does not tell us the causal direction of this association. One interpretation may forward the argument, that risk-taking propensity may have an influence on decision making in terms of sleep, thus lowering sleep duration. It may as well be the other way around—lack of sleep fosters risky decisions. On the other hand, both sleep and risk behavior may be impacted by third variables like family environment or parental limit setting [10]. In conclusion, it is most likely that the elucidation of causal relationships still deserves further studies. If sleep loss in the end leads to more risky decision making and increases levels of risk-taking behavior, this may start a self-perpetuating cycle, with poor sleep leading to poor decision making about sleep, leading to poorer sleep and so on [10]. In this respect, a risk escalation may occur.

2.3.1 Internet Addiction, Problematic Media Use and the "Invisible Risk Group"

In today's society, almost everyone has open access to the internet around the clock, whether through their computer, smartphone or tablet. With the spread of the internet, related problems of the "darknet"—like pornography and criminal activities—have increased significantly in the last two decades as well as personal risks, such as pathological internet usage [70]. Since the phenomenon of pathological internet use particularly affects adolescents, extensive research into the associated problems and triggering factors is an important task of today's research in risk behaviors [71, 72]. The term "pathological internet use" is often also referred to as internet addiction. In this respect it seems important to differentiate pathological internet use that fulfills the criteria of addiction from excessive media and internet consumption without addiction criteria. Internet addiction itself comprises addiction to various online activities, which can be reduced to five categories according to Young et al. [73]: online games, social media, internet pornography, gambling and online research.

After a long and controversial debate, the "Internet Gaming Disorder" was included in the research appendix (conditions for further study) of the Diagnostic and Statistical Manual of Mental Disorders, Fifth Edition (DSM-5) [74]. The criteria of this disorder have been developed based on those for substance-related addictions and include preoccupation, withdrawal symptoms, development of tolerance, loss of control over participation in games, loss of interests, continuation despite negative consequences, dysfunctional stress management to relieve negative mood, dissimulation and deception of family members regarding the amount of gaming, jeopardized and lost relationships [74]. In the new International Classification of Diseases, 11th Edition (ICD-11) of the World Health Organization (WHO), the disorder, broader than computer and internet addiction, will be listed in the chapter on behavioral addictions.

41.3% of adolescents in the United States spent more than 3 h online not dedicated to school work on school days (overview [75]). The prevalence figures for pathological internet use reported so far show a high degree of variance ranging from 0.2% up to 34% depending on different countries [75]. According to current surveys, a prevalence of around 4.4% can be assumed in Europe [76]. However, there is a clear trend that the prevalence of internet addiction increases with the spread of internet access [70]. Within the subcategories of internet addiction, girls have a higher prevalence of dependency on social media, while internet game addiction in turn shows a higher incidence among boys [77].

The review by Maria von Salisch [78] on violent computer games questions the myth of the direct causation of aggression by computer games, which is repeatedly tried in the trivial literature. Even if there is a socialization effect from violent computer games, which stems from working with such games and can intensify physical aggression in adolescents, this effect remains weak with a beta value of 0.11 and shrinks completely to a beta of 0.08 if explanatory third variables—such as gender and social class—are included [79]. The examination of selection effects (aggressive individuals prefer aggressive games) reveals that these appear more clearly in larger samples and at the beginning of adolescence. Interventions at the beginning of adolescence appear to be particularly successful. Encountering friends still remains the number one leisure activity and the occupation with computer games is currently in fourth place.

Another problem behavior comprises pornography use of adolescents. There is clear evidence of a negative impact on social interaction and bonding, lower life satisfaction and lower satisfaction with sexual experiences, besides a negative effect on self-esteem [80]. Pornography depicts fleeting sexual encounters that are devoid of intimacy and prolonged exposure may disrupt the development of healthy relationship styles and impair social functioning [80]. In Croatia, a group of adolescents with 1287 participants was assessed with a mean age of 15.9 years. In female adolescents' higher initial frequency of pornography use was related to more anxiety and depression symptoms and lower self-esteem at baseline. No significant associations were detected between pornography use and well-being indicators among male participants. Latent growth trajectory classes revealed no significant correspondence between growth in pornography use and changes in the well-being indicators in both sexes [80] over 30 months. However, the long-term effects on self-objectification and social scripts still wait to be elucidated empirically.

Smartphone use has become widespread amongst adolescents. Do these data parallel the increases of poor mental health in this group? The existence of a smartphone addiction and problematic smartphone use is discussed under the headline of media concern [81]. In a meta-analysis of 924 studies on problematic smartphone use and mental health outcome, more than 41,000 children and adolescents were included. The median prevalence of problematic smartphone use was 23.3%. For this group increased odds of depression, higher anxiety scores, more perceived stress and poorer sleep quality were documented [81]. Problematic phone use may be an evolving public concern that requires greater attention to determine the boundary between helpful and harmful technology use in adolescents [81].

The "invisible-risk group" (29% of adolescents) in the European study [69] who scored positive for high use of internet/TV/videogames, sedentary behavior and reduced sleep seem to be of special interest. In this group adolescent sleep deprivation may be a matter of increased concern. Although socially quiet, this group may develop psychopathological features and emotional secondary problems in the same way as the socially conspicuous risk group. A disruption of the adolescent's circadian clock may have several neuroendocrine and behavioral consequences [75].

2.3.2   Substance Abuse (Alcohol and Drugs), Smoking and Tobacco Use

Problem behavior theory asserts that delinquency and other risky behaviors like substance abuse form a set of problematic behavior, which in its core reflects a detachment from convention [82]. Normal adolescent's detachment from convention in the sense of a search for one's own leeway may be accentuated or disrupted by traumatic childhood experiences in the individual biography. Youth with the history of childhood sexual abuse may be especially vulnerable for such interferences [83]. Early adolescent substance use and abuse as a risky experiment for unusual experiences may dramatically increase the risk for lifelong substance use disorder [84]. Early substance use—whether of legal substances or illicit drugs—interferes with ongoing neurodevelopment to induce functional changes that further may augment the risk of substance use disorder. It is hypothesized that an immature prefrontal cortex combined with hyper-reactivity of reward salience and stress-reaction may lead to increased vulnerability [84]. Changes of sleep and circadian misalignment may impair the reward related brain mechanisms and thus increase the risk of alcohol use disorders. [75]. On the other hand, alcohol itself is able to desynchronize the circadian system. The adolescent brain—especially the hippocampus—may be particularly vulnerable to the effects of alcohol predisposing the adolescent to neurocognitive problems that may persist into adulthood [85]. Adolescent binge drinking has become increasingly common among teenagers. The age peak can be determined between 18 and 25 years. However, in the age group 14 to 16 years in Europe the prevalence of consuming alcohol 2–3 days per week could be documented in 13.4%, with significantly higher rates observed in males compared to females [67]. The harmful effects of exposure to radical marketing strategies for alcohol products in our society should be underlined [75].

Tobacco use is started and established in adolescence. The prevalence of smoking in European adolescents is relatively high with 30.9% [67]. Onset was reported before the age of 14 years. In the SEYLE-study on students in the age between 14 and 16 years smoking was significantly associated with emotional problems, conduct problems, hyperactivity, excessive alcohol and illicit drug use and previous suicide attempts [86]. Although cigarette use by adolescents has declined in recent years in most western countries, around 21% of US youth ages 12 to 17 years have tried a tobacco product. 13% tried traditional cigarettes, 11% electronic cigarettes, 8% cigars and 4% smokeless tobacco [87]. Digital media provide increased opportunities for both marketing and social transmission of risky products and behavior [88]. Waterpipe smoking has become increasingly interesting for young people as a product of globalization. It is known to be harmful to health. Estimates of use prevalence for adults in Europe unexpectedly seem equally high compared to eastern countries [89]. Electronic cigarettes as relatively new devices could form a gateway for starting tobacco use in young people. 1.9% of 14 to 17 years old youngsters use electronic cigarettes in Germany. 74.5% of them also smoke tobacco in the sense of a dual use [90].

Although around three-fourth of American adolescents do not think there may be a great risk in using cannabis, it has to be pointed out that there is a strong association between early frequent and heavy cannabis exposure in adolescence with impaired cognition and an adverse neuropsychiatric outcome in adulthood [75]. There is an increased risk for the development of depression and schizophrenia. In their paper, Denisa Ghinea and the Heidelberg research group [91] investigated the relationship between drug use and symptoms of borderline disorder in patients of a special outpatient clinic for risk behaviors. 347 adolescents (81.7% female) were examined. Results showed that the symptoms of borderline syndrome in adolescents are clearly associated with drug use. There was no difference with regard to occasional or regular consumption. However, regular drug users were more impulsive and more often affected by uncontrolled anger. Regarding the symptom of depression, no systematic correlations with drug use could be detected in the patient group.

2.3.3   Non-Suicidal Self-Injury (NSSI) and Suicidal Behavior

There are undoubtedly differences between today's body staging's, instrumentalizations and self-optimizations of the body of youth in comparison with earlier youth cultures, especially in terms of the dynamics and radicalism of the reification and objectification of one's own body. Self-harm and self-mutilations as symptoms of disturbances in self-development in adolescents have attracted increasing attention in recent years. Self-harm has a paradoxical function of self-care. Non-suicidal self-injury (NSSI)—which is the most actual term for self-mutilation—may reduce unbearable tensions, allow urgent suicide ideas to take a back seat and interrupt the fear of self-loss and a feeling of "going crazy". From a biographical point of view, childhood traumas including sexual abuse experiences may be frequently detected, which are mostly based on profound emotional neglect in early relationships [58]. The basic motives of self-regulation and self-presentation are identified by two patient self-reports: "When I no longer feel myself, I cut myself and realize that I'm still alive." (quote from a 16-year-old patient). "If something hurts me terribly inside, then I hurt myself so that you can see how much it hurts me." (quote from a 15-year-old patient).

In young people, the overall frequency of self-harming behavior is not evenly distributed between the genders. We observe the behavior in girls much more often than in boys. It appears that the gender difference is even more pronounced in adolescence than in later adulthood [58]. In older studies, a ratio of 2:1 to 9:1 for female patients has been described [92]. In recent studies, the prevalence of the female gender is two to three times higher (2–3:1) than that of the male [93]. In our Heidelberg school study, the gender difference in self-harming behavior was 2:1 for girls, but in repetitive self-harming behavior, the gender ratio was characterized by a female preponderance of 3:1 [94]. The reasons for these gender differences are always interpreted differently. Some argue that teenage girls are more irritable and appear rather fearful and depressive. Other causes are seen in increased interpersonal conflicts in the adolescence phase. The idea that the female gender may tend to show more auto-aggressive behavior, while the male gender tends to act out emotional problems through outward destructive behavior may—although fitting the epidemiological data—rather be a story of clichéd myths, especially when biological explanations of hormonal differences are applied. Since, as has been shown, self-harming behaviors are associated with psychological traumas in the biography, the increased self-harming behaviors in girls could be an alarming sign of increased psychological injuries in women [95].

The distinction between self-harming behavior and suicidal behavior—which makes death and dying the essential content of the intended action—appears to be of particular importance. In contrast, self-harming behaviors have a paradoxical function of self-care: Especially with urgent suicide ideas and strong suicide impulses, the implementation of self-harming behaviors (e.g. making cuts on the forearm) can reduce the unbearable tension so that suicidal intentions can be reduced. Self-injuring acts in NSSI do therefore not represent unsuccessful suicide attempts, but can have an almost auto-protective character [96]. In research literature, however, opinions on the relationship between suicidality and self-harming behavior are quite controversial [58]. In particular, there is a different intention with self-harming behaviors, which accepts death but does not make it the central goal of action [97]. Epidemiologically, however, we find a strong association between the frequency of self-injurious behavior and suicidality. Almost 50% of adolescents who injure themselves more than 5 times a year have attempted suicide several

times. NSSI appears to be a time-invariant predictor of adolescent suicide ideation
and suicide attempts in a diverse community sample [98] and suicide related behaviors have been linked to reactive aggression [99]. Studies support the idea of a specific distress-function relationship in adolescent NSSI [100]. In a representative
clinical sample engagement with NSSI was significantly related to adverse childhood experiences with highest associations for maternal antipathy and neglect [101].

What are the behavioral intentions and motives for NSSI? In a study conducted
to explore possible motives for self-harm in 65 inpatients [101], a three-factor model
was detected in the factor analysis of the interview data, reflecting the clinical situation quite well. A factor of "intrapsychic functions"—in the sense of self-regulation,
evidence to be alive and cut down feelings of tension—had to be differentiated from
a factor with "interpersonal interaction" effects. These motives tried to show the
others one's own problems and involve the environment into the personal conflicts.
A third factor, called "peer-identification", recorded the phenomena that we may
also name as group contagion effects of self-harm. It included mainly feelings of
belonging, self-enhancement, recognition and participation in the peer group.

NSSI are strongly related to environmental stress and present with a course of
self-limitation. However, in a longitudinal study we were able to show that risky
alcohol use and maintenance of self-injurious behavior remained as significant pre-
dictors of borderline personality development in a stepwise binomial regression [102].

The following data should convey the importance of differentiating between risk
behavior and psychopathology: A representative sample of 5759 ninth-grade students was studied. Deliberate self-harm, suicidality and emotional and behavioral
problems were assessed. There appeared to be a link between school-related and
family-related social problems and occasional self-harm, in repetitive self-harm a
strong association with suicidal behavior as well as emotional and behavioral problems could be detected [94]. Different pathways seem to exist in the development of
deliberate self-harm. Occasional acts of self-mutilation seem to represent a transient
period of stress, while repetitive self-injurious behavior indicates deeper psychiatric
disturbances. Frequency and intensity of non-suicidal self-injury indicate the severity of an accompanying mental disturbance. Patients of an outpatient service presenting with self-injury as a stand-alone diagnosis seem to be rare and associated
with low illness severity and less psychopathological distress compared with
patients with higher psychiatric comorbidity [103]. Risk behaviors indicate and promote mental problems, their intensity reflects the problem pressure and the degree
of overwhelming.

2.3.4   Disordered Eating and Diets

Eating disorders are of high clinical and social relevance. They are among the most
common chronic mental disturbances in adulthood with a high incidence and a disease peak already in adolescence. Eating disorders are often associated with serious

consequences, such as exploding costs of the welfare system, acute and chronic concomitant diseases or school- and professional failure [104]. 19.8% of children and adolescents in an epidemiological survey of the Robert Koch Institute addressing health aspects in 6599 German youngsters show symptoms of an eating disorder. This is a decrease of 2.8 percentage points compared to 10 years ago. This decline particularly affects 11- to 13-year-old boys, while the risk for 14- to 17-year-olds and especially for girls has remained comparably high. Children and adolescents with emotional problems, low family cohesion or low self-efficacy have an increased risk for developing symptoms of eating disorders [104]. Another risk factor seems to be the body image perception. Body image distortions such as perception bias have been detected in 11–17 years old boys and girls. There is a systematic underestimation in the judgement of the average body size of young women on naturalistic photographs [105]. Girls and boys generally held a slim female thin-ideal. A substantial proportion displayed an underweight thin-ideal (24.9% among girls, 16.8% among boys). Early adolescent girls (13–14 years) presented with the strongest thin-ideal internalization. Symptoms of disturbed eating, e.g. harmful dieting behavior and psychological stress associated with eating were reported frequently in those girls with a body image perception bias and an underweight thin-ideal [105].

Several risk factors for eating disorders can be detected in numerous studies: female gender, thin-ideal internalization, low self- esteem and adverse interpersonal experiences [106]. The most widely studied cultural theory is objectification theory. In cultures, where the female body is objectified and seen as a tool for sexual pleasure or gratification to men, girls and women are at increased risk of eating disorders. Mechanisms like self-objectification, thin-ideal internalization, body shame and body surveillance mediate this process [106]. Cultural pressure to achieve a thin beauty ideal increases the risk for eating disorders across gender groups. Family and peer pressure about appearance were significantly associated with risk for anorexia or bulimia [106].

Individual factors of self-esteem and narcissistic control seem to have an impact on dieting behavior and eating problems. It seems that "hiding the self"—an unwillingness to show one's faults and needs to others—may lead to the idea of extreme control over emotions, needs and relations. These self-aspects may contribute to the development of eating disorders [107].

2.3.5 Adolescent Aggression, Violence and Delinquency

The development lines, preliminary stages and courses of physical aggression patterns could be defined and clarified in many studies [108]. Physical aggression begins in kindergarten and toddler age. It seems to gradually decrease over the school age years into adolescence. However, there is a group of children who remain physically aggressive through adolescence until adulthood. The genders are not distributed equally in different course groups. Almost two times the number of boys as girls exhibit physical aggression during childhood and adolescence. The chronically aggressive group from childhood to adolescence contains many more boys than girls [109].

In addition, a concept of indirect aggression is defined. It is a more covert and interpersonal form of aggression. It manifests itself above all through social manipulation: spreading rumors, acting behind the backs of others, or asking others to avoid or to target people. Physical conflicts and open violence are avoided. Indirect aggression also begins with preschool age and then usually remains stable at a low level. In some individuals, there is a marked increase in these behaviors as they progress into adolescence. There are significantly more girls in this cohort [109]. The literature confirms that physical aggression and indirect aggression are moderately correlated across different ages.

In the Canadian study, which examined both forms of aggression in combination [109], it was possible to investigate forms of progression from pre-puberty to adolescence to emergent adult. The developmental courses between the ages of 10 and 19 were traced in more than 2.300 children of a representative sample. Three groups of developmental trajectories of physical aggression could be modeled over three measuring points over the age of 10 to 15 years: 32.5% showed no physical aggression. A group of moderate aggression with a decreasing tendency comprised 52.2%, a group with high still increasing aggression level comprised 15.3%. In this study, too, the higher levels of physical aggression were more linked to the male sex.

Similar courses of between 10 and 15 years were found for indirect aggression. a low-declining group comprised 29.9%. A moderate group with a decreasing course comprised 65.5%, while a highly stable group comprised 4.6%. Examination of the joint association of physical and indirect aggression showed that about half of the adolescents were in a moderate, declining group that included both forms of aggression. A group with low indirect aggression without physical aggression comprised 20% of the study participants. Only 7% had high levels of physical and indirect aggression.

It can be seen that both forms of aggression develop similarly over age and that increases in one form of aggression were accompanied by increases in the other. It was shown that the adolescents, whose course was linked to high indirect aggression and high-increasing trajectories of physical aggression, or to moderate indirect aggression and high-increasing trajectories of physical aggression, showed significantly higher rates of mismatch with the environment and maladjustment in emergent adulthood when compared with the group with low indirect aggression without physical aggression [109].

It has to be assumed that there is a kind of dose-response relationship to accumulating risks [110]. Increased risk factors in different areas of life across multiple domains increase the likelihood of later unfavorable courses. Increased dissocial and aggressive behavior can be expected leading to adverse outcomes e.g. delinquency.

Aggression turns out to be a risk factor for the development of persistent delinquent behavior. The influential taxonomic theory developed by Moffitt [111] stated that two qualitatively distinct profiles in delinquent offenders can be distinguished.

One is of a life-persistent character and comprises around 5–8% of the general population. Individuals exhibit antisocial behavior since childhood and continue to show this behavior through adolescence into adulthood [112]. The other profile is called "adolescence-limited" and comprises a rather common group with antisocial behavior restricted to the adolescent phase. However, this taxonomy has been critically reviewed on the basis of empirical evidence [113]. There are children with severe antisocial traits in childhood who desist from this behavior during adolescence showing that there is no fateful course of these behavioral traits. On the other hand, not all delinquent behaviors starting later in adolescence seem to be limited to this phase and can persist into adulthood. Both profiles seem to resemble each other in terms of risk factors leading to the conclusion that the distinction between them is rather quantitative—pertaining to the number of antecedents, than qualitative—pertaining to the nature of antecedents [112]. Multiple risk domains have been identified. The review of Assink et al. [112] meta-analytically summarized the data of 55 studies from 1995 to 2014. The total sample consisted of 13,872 juveniles, 4596 persistent offenders and 9276 limited offenders. 14 domains of risk factors were included: Criminal history, aggression, alcohol and drug abuse, sexual risk behavior, relationship patterns, emotional problems, school/employment problems, family problems, neurocognitive deficits, attitudes, physical health, neighborhood and several others. Cohen's d was calculated to express the effect of a risk factor for life-course-persistent offending relative to adolescent-limited offending. The strongest effects were found in the criminal history and aggression domains. Levels of risk factors were significantly higher in most domains in the life-persistent offender group. It can be concluded, that multiple risk domains are involved in delinquent behavior, and that the difference between life-time persistent and adolescent-limited behavior is rather quantitative than qualitative [112]. The extent of unfavorable living conditions and life events seems to shape the course of delinquent behavior, not any innate willingness or genetic vulnerability.

A new analysis of longitudinal data with structural MRI showed 672 participants out of a cohort of 1037 individuals born between April 1972 and March 1973. The study revealed differences in brain morphometry associated with life-time persistent antisocial behavior [114]. These differences in surface areas and cortical thickness between participants with low antisocial activities and the lifetime persistent antisocial group again do not sustain simple theories of a genetic trait for antisocial behavior, because the brain maps life-time experiences and behavioral adaptation within structural network development. Brain structures and functions do not exclusively "cause" behavior. Brain plasticity reflects the brain networks and their structures to be shaped by experience and behavior. Brain architecture and function reflect biographical history.

2.3.6   Sexual Risk Behavior: Sexually Transmitted Diseases and Adolescent Pregnancy

Sexual risk behavior is defined as the exchange of sexual acts or practices by an individual in exchange for commodities, such as food, shelter, money or drugs—including sex work (prostitution) as a form of "survival sex" [115]. Other definitions include all forms of unprotected sex with sexual random partners with the increased risk for sexually transmitted diseases or sexual offences and traumatization. Childhood sexual abuse may have an indirect effect on risky sexual behavior by externalizing problems. This pattern is equally valid for boys and girls [83].

Sexually transmitted diseases constitute a major health problem affecting mostly young people not only in the developing countries, but also in Western and European countries [116]. Although during the 80s of the last century a decrease of most sexually transmitted diseases had been observed, from the mid-90s on a new increase in syphilis, gonorrhea and chlamydia have been reported in several European countries for the age group of 16–19 years old [116]. If these diseases occur symptom-free they can be passed on unaware during unprotected intercourse. Although knowledge and awareness are known to be of limited effect on changing attitudes and behaviors, they seem to be important components of sex education which help promote informed choices in adolescents. A review comprising 15 studies tried to focus on awareness and knowledge of sexually transmitted diseases in school attending adolescents [116]. The highest awareness and knowledge were reported for HIV/AIDS. More than 90% of the individuals asked were able to identify the disease as a sexually transmitted disease. More than 80% identified gonorrhea from a list of diseases, awareness of syphilis was surveyed in England, where 45% of adolescents correctly identified this disease. 56% in another study identified herpes correctly as a sexually transmitted disease. The lowest identification rates were reported for HPV (human papilloma virus), with awareness as low as 5.4% in one study [116]. The awareness may increase since the introduction of the HPV-vaccine. Gender also appears to have an influence on awareness of sexually transmitted diseases, especially for HPV. Significant gender differences were observed, with females having better awareness and knowledge than males [116].

A systematic review investigating substance use in its association with sexual risk behaviors and sexual victimization identified and reviewed 23 studies [115]. It was shown that substance abuse was associated with sexual risk behavior or sexual victimization. However, it remains unclear whether substance use preceded or followed sexual behaviors and experiences. But one has to assume that the interaction of risky sexual behavior and drug use can lead to escalating cycles of individual risk. Homeless youth, in particular, experience various forms of sexual victimization witnessing and fearing the sexual behavior of others [115].

Teen pregnancy continues to be another major area of concern not only in Europe. Teen pregnancy places the adolescent mother at multiple risks like low educational attainment, unemployment or poverty [117]. On the other hand, teen mothers are also at an increased risk for adverse pregnancy outcomes, e.g. eclampsia, preterm delivery, low birth weight, and neonatal complications [117]. The prevalence of postpartum depression among adolescent mothers is significantly higher compared to adult mothers [118]. This is of importance, because postpartum depression does not only affect the young women, but has also an impact on the development of the child [119]. Higher levels of maternal depression are associated with greater developmental delays in infants at 18 months of age [120]. Another area of concern is the prevention of repeat pregnancy in adolescents. Approximately 35% of recently pregnant adolescents have experienced a rapid repeat pregnancy, most of which (around two thirds) were unintended [118]. Prevention of pregnancy is the first-line approach as most teen pregnancies appear to be unplanned. This comprises comprehensive sex education and counseling on contraception [118]. Data indicate that rates of teen pregnancy have declined in the last decade, which is likely the result of a combination of a decline in sexual activity and increased contraceptive use and efficacy [121]. Offering highly effective contraception to adolescents may help decrease the number of teen pregnancies and avoid adverse outcomes [117].

2.3.7 Bullying, School Stress and School Absenteeism

Bullying in schools has gained increasing attention during the last years. Violence and failure to respect human limits, physical injury and blackmail in school represents a serious social problem. Prevalence rates for school bullying vary greatly depending on the definition used. In a large-scale study comprising 40 different countries, Craig et al. [122] concluded that approx. 13% of the students were detected as victims, 11% as perpetrators and 4% as bully/victims. The bullying rates of the individual countries varied considerably. The pressure of suffering from school bullying is enormous, the risk for emotional disorders and behavioral problems increases significantly on both the victim and the perpetrator side, including impaired school development and decreased academic achievement for both sides. The relationship between bullying and depression, suicidality and self-injurious behavior has been addressed in a study with 303 pupils of whom 20.8% said they had been a victim of bullying in the past few months. The emotional problems—depression, suicidality and self-injurious behavior—were shown to be significantly increased for victimized students (odds ratios from 2.4 to 3.0) [123]. Prevention programs are needed to stop this trend [124].

Problems related to school attendance are also common [52]. Frequent school absenteeism has not only immediate effects on academic performance, but also on long term social functioning, high school and college graduation rates, adult income, health and life expectancy [125]. School absenteeism therefore represents a public health issue and an educational problem involving mental health professionals, physicians, teachers, and educators [126]. Prevalence rates for problematic school absenteeism in Europe are estimated to be as high as 5–10%. Up to 30% of affected students suffer from mental health problems [52]. In the USA a recent national survey found that even 14% of students—from kindergarten to the 12th grade—are chronically absent, defined as missing at least 10% of the school year (estimated as 18 days) with a high variance between the districts from less than 5% up to 50%! [125]. Factors associated with higher risk of chronic absenteeism on the individual level comprise chronic somatic illness, bullying, and other risk behaviors like substance abuse, exposure to aggression, sleep deficiency, and mental health problems. Family factors of caregiving, health problems of family members, lack of structure and supervision, social risk factors and parent unemployment are of equal importance. However, there are also school and community factors increasing the risk of absenteeism: cultural barriers, economic disadvantage, poor social climate, unsafe neighborhood, or being a member of a socially vulnerable group like bisexuality or transgender [125]. A meta-analysis of 75 studies reporting on 781 potential risk factors for school absenteeism revealed risk domains with large effects including a negative attitude towards school, substance abuse, externalizing and internalizing mental problems of the juvenile and a low parent-school involvement [127]. Prevention, intervention and therapy should be performed in a stepped care manner with a multimodal and multi-systemic approach [128]. Creating networks of help will be of higher importance than systematic medical interventions alone.

2.4   Conclusion: The Functional Aspect

Risk behaviors form a set of behaviors that are not primarily caused by disease processes! However, they may turn out to be triggers of or partly accompanying psychological disorders. As DiClemente et al. [51] state: "Many adolescents today, and perhaps an increasing number in the future, are at risk for death, disease, and other adverse health outcomes that are not primarily biomedical in origin … At present, however, the overwhelming toll of adolescent morbidity and mortality is the result of life practices." These behaviors—potentially preventable in nature—may be the result of overwhelming adaptation processes due to the complexities of the postmodern world and the task of becoming adults in this particular world (see Chap. 10).

As risk behaviors are more likely to be endemic among adolescents—compared to children or adults [10]—it is imperative to understand factors that may help mitigate at least some of the detrimental consequences thereof. Risk behaviors present with a fundamental functional aspect. They serve the self and its regulation. They serve the adaptation processes and make fundamental sense to the individual for the moment, however, they may cause damage, harm, suffering, and death in the long run. The adolescents will always stick to such behaviors until these can be replaced by suitable alternative behaviors. To provide help in this sense means to get an understanding of the functional properties of these behaviors. Help by alternatives can only be offered, if there is an understanding of the adaptive functions of risk behaviors and symptoms. Risk behaviors may represent precursors of more serious mental disorders, and in the worst case can also turn into those disorders of a disease nature. However, the starting point is always the lifestyle-behavior [59], triggered by environmental circumstances.

Chapter 3
Developmental Psychopathology and Emotional Regulation

3.1 Definitions

Developmental psychopathology ambitiously provides an overview of the unfolding knowledge on mental disorders and the variety of therapeutic approaches available in a new synopsis by integrating clinical developmental psychological knowledge and psychiatric experience into a bio-psycho-social model [129, 130]. Developmental psychopathology is therefore concerned not only with the pathogenesis of mental disorders, but also in particular with the clinical course over the further lifespan. Clinical decisions will be therapeutically enriched through the application of developmental psychological knowledge. The development focus is directed to different areas: on the one hand, the influences of normal development on the genesis and manifestation of psychopathological symptoms in different ages are considered, on the other hand, the influence of psychopathological symptoms on normal development is the subject of the study [129]. In different phases of life children typically have very different ways of reacting to mental irritation. The infant's forms of expression of distress focus mainly on changes in eating, sleeping, and excretion behavior, and the interactional alarm situation, in which the child uses crying to make the caregiver aware of his or her condition. The different forms of fear, for example, separation anxiety, dark fear, social anxiety or fear of existence are also tied to important cognitive developmental steps of the child and adolescent. We also know that toddlers may not develop delusions as long as they cannot take social perspectives. Delusions need the takeover of another's focus. We expect social perspectives to be adopted by children from the age of four earliest.

Developmental Psychopathology is based on developmental theories, which we call "interactionist", whereby we assume that an active, self-motivated individual who intentionally drives his own development interacts with an equally active, demanding and influencing environment [129]. The human psyche is not a "tabula

F. Resch, P. Parzer, *Adolescent Risk Behavior and Self-Regulation*,
https://doi.org/10.1007/978-3-030-69955-0_3

rasa"—an empty wax panel—where life events are going to be inscribed, equally the psychological processes do not unfold solely as the result of inborn mechanisms without being shaped by the surrounding.

The emotional dialogue with important caregivers and the socio-cultural influences of the environment—which go beyond the family—have a framing and shaping character. However, the children are not simply at the mercy of these influences; rather, they play an active role in shaping this environment themselves: we can assume that the child influences its environmental conditions as actively and shapes them in the same way as it is influenced by these external conditions. If developmental psychopathology wants to examine the causal conditions and the course of individual patterns of mismatches in child and adolescent development, it must always focus on the specific problems of adaptation to environmental demands and the coping endeavors with developmental needs [131–135].

3.2   Models of Developmental Psychopathology

In addition to the interactionist developmental theory already mentioned, the issues of risks and resources, vulnerabilities and resilience play a fundamental role for the understanding of mental health problems [130]. Psychopathological phenomena are examined more closely in terms of their adaptation value and have to be related to developmental tasks in each age group. The functionality of psychopathological symptoms and the individual developmental influences will be discussed in detail below (Chap. 6).

3.2.1   Developmental Tasks

It should be emphasized that in the perspective of developmental psychopathology, a therapeutic influence on dysfunctionality and suffering can never lead back to a virtual starting point of normality, in the sense of a cure from insane to sane, but that favorable therapeutic processes bring symptoms to an end and change the direction of behavior into a frame of higher functionality so that normal developmental processes get the upper hand. Normality is therefore not a static term, not a state of homeostasis, but a reference area of a favorable future-oriented developmental process.

Adaptation is shown not only as a confrontation with adverse environmental influences, but also as a functional coping with developmental tasks [23]. Such developmental tasks are age-typical challenges that every human individual has to face. For example, building relationships with important caregivers in early childhood is not only a cultural challenge, but also a biologically necessary and socially desirable developmental task (see Chap. 1). Havighurst [23] described a series of bio-psycho-social development steps, which must be successfully mastered as developmental tasks. This coping ultimately leads to skills and competencies which in turn make mastering future developmental tasks easier. In addition to more biologically determined developmental tasks such as learning to stand and walk, there are also tasks that are primarily socio-cultural, such as school challenges of learning to read and write. We assume that the successful mastering of developmental tasks is the basis for a smooth development and for mental well-being [129]. If developmental tasks are not mastered, this can lead to complications for the further developmental steps and to a mismatch in the adaptation processes. The symptoms of a disorder, in turn, can have an adaptive function in relation to the developmental tasks themselves [129]. Symptoms may be a way of trying to cope with being overwhelmed (see Chap. 7).

3.2.2 Risks and Protective Factors

While risks are a burden on a child's development, resources are characterized by protective factors. Risk factors are defined by life events and external influences, which in children increase the likelihood of a developmental deviation or disruption [132]. Such risks can be primarily biologically effective—e.g. through premature birth or cerebral inflammatory processes—or through special psychological experiences of social deprivation or drastic events, such as the death of a caregiver. Some risk factors, such as drug-abuse, affect both the biological and psychosocial areas. Risk factors not only increase the likelihood of suffering, development of symptoms, and ultimately illness, but also make adaptation more difficult. Risk factors can also prevent developmental tasks from being accomplished. Risk factors themselves are not a static variable, but rather have a process-related influence on the development. In contrast, protective factors are to be understood as part of the resources, they are often thought to be complementary to the risk factors: while negative communication in the family is a risk factor, a positive family climate can be seen as a protective factor. Protective factors reduce the effects of risks, they promote the management of development tasks and help to compensate for unfavorable influences. Protective factors open up new opportunities. An interplay between development risks and protective factors is to be noted in such a way that if there are too many risky influences, positive influences by protective factors can no longer be observed. It therefore appears that protective factors can mitigate individual risks, but that their influence is weakened under massive risk conditions [136]. We may assume that the number of risk factors that a child is exposed to is of specific importance. Not (only) the type, but rather the number of risk factors have a negative developmental impact.

3.2.3 Vulnerability and Resilience

The basic concept for the development of risk behaviors and mental disturbances is the vulnerability model. As a dynamic concept, it can be clearly distinguished from a genetic determination model. Vulnerability can be accentuated by innate factors, but it itself has to be understood in terms of the process. Vulnerability thus proves to be viable and only potentially relevant for disruption, while the genetic influences may in any case impair further development. Special vulnerabilities can actually give rise to compensatory processes for higher and further developments [129]. In contrast, the genetic defect has a negative impact on all developmental phases and increases the risk of psychological decompensation. We therefore define vulnerability as a particular sensitivity to negative environmental conditions, so that vulnerability only really comes into effect under risk conditions (see Fig. 3.1).

In contrast, we describe resilience as a person's particular withstanding to stressful circumstances [137, 138]. This refers to those children who develop favorably despite extreme risk conditions. Resilience can not only be measured by the level of performance that is maintained despite adverse circumstances, it must also include aspects of life satisfaction and well-being in a complex form. Resilience itself is the result of a complex adaptation and developmental process and not a purely innate personality trait. Resilience is acquired by the child in interaction with its environment during the course of development [132]. No one can develop resilience in all domains of life because resilience is not a lasting, stable and all-encompassing ability. There are many more situation-specific and context-dependent resilience processes that have to be viewed as parameters [130].

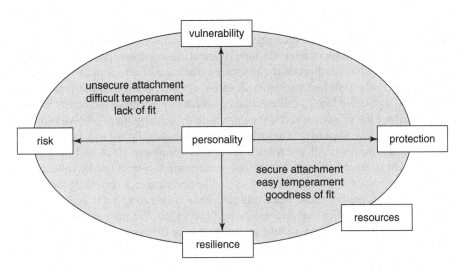

Fig. 3.1 Developmental spaces of childhood

Three tenets of resilience were finally defined [139]:

- *Plasticity* implicates the flexible adaptation to changing conditions. It comprises the ability to integrate and calibrate various subcomponents, e.g. self-regulation or parent-child co-regulation.
- *Sociality* means the ability for cooperation and coordinated action to enhance the survival of the group. Bonding confers resilience by supporting the maturation of stress-management systems, providing protection and ushering social collaboration.
- *Meaning-making systems* sustain resilience. They give significance to human suffering and inspire strength in the face of trauma. Death may be transcended through acts of kindness.

3.2.4 The Emotional System

One of the key assumptions of developmental psychopathology is that the understanding of emotional processes is fundamental for the understanding of risk behaviors and psychopathological phenomena. In the sense of an "affective turn", which behavioral sciences have recorded since the late 1990s, affective decision-making and evaluation processes are particularly used to explain psychological problems in addition to the cognitive explanation models. Affects are innate, psychological reaction patterns that have developed from reflex and instinctual programs in the course of phylogenetic brain development [129, 140]. Both the expression components and the experience components of affective states are subsumed under the concept of emotion. Emotions thus represent an extension of the concept of affects into the field of cognitive information processing. Affects and their cognitive awareness-processes form the basis of emotions. While basic affective tones remain relatively constant over the lifespan, expressive (mimic) components, cognitive evaluations and decision-making are addressed as age-related development processes.

Affects create an acute need for action in the subject; urgency is created. The entire repertoire of behavior is available for the response. This means that affects versus reflexes are a phylogenetic advantage, since there is no longer a fixed link between the stimulus and the response, but additional degrees of freedom of action are provided if the individual can respond to their situational triggers with different planned actions under affect pressure. As affective-cognitive processes, emotions represent a superordinate, close-to-the-body decision-making system that not only signals urgency internally and initiates appropriate patterns of action, but also expresses the inner state of mind through interaction with other people. Emotional expressions in facial expressions, gestures and words are legible and understandable and thus form the basis of the emotional dialogue that comes to develop between the mother—as well as any caregiver—and the child, long before the child learns to speak, as an interpersonal relationship. Facial communication has a signal effect that is also used in relationship regulation [141]. The emotional dialogue forms the natural basis for the phenomenon of intersubjectivity.

From birth, children have different abilities to deal with intense feelings. The basis of emotional regulation is therefore a constitutional disposition, which is also expressed in different temperament characteristics. Children have different abilities to regulate their emotional states from birth. However, this regulation of the infant's condition cannot be understood purely from a somatic point of view. Because, right from the start, affective regulation is influenced by an interactional component of relationships with important caregivers [142]. By perceiving parental affects, infants can resonance the emotional state which the parents express nonverbally (see overview [30]). Even newborns react to the cries of other newborns with screams, we refer to such phenomena as contagion. It remains to be seen whether facial expressions play a special role in the process of affective resonance—so that imitation creates a similar emotion in the child to that of the caregiver. The inner state of parents does not only appear to be reflected in their facial expression, it can also be demonstrated by other physiological parameters e.g. voice tone, heart-beat or muscular tension [30].

Affect resonance can have both calming and worrying effects in children. The calming effect of affect attunement has been described by Stern [143]. In this way, facial expressions of the parents can not only directly reflect their own emotional state, but the parents are also able to express their thoughts and inner ideas in their facial expressions in a symbolic way when dealing with their child. In this way, facial expressions can convey and make available to the other party particular information that go beyond their own status report. The caregivers can, in particular, reflect the child's emotional state in their own facial expressions and thus symbolically convey the child's emotions. This process is called social bio-feedback. This phenomenon, originally described by Gergely and Watson, was finally conceptualized further by Fonagy in collaboration with the authors mentioned [144]. Affect mirroring enables parents to accentuate the utterances of the infant and, in a playful way, influence the child's affects in interaction with the children—in the sense of co-regulation. For example, a short smile on the child's face can be deliberately grasped and mimicked by the parents, so that the infant is made aware of their own condition: a process of socio-emotional biofeedback is started [144]. The infant recognizes that information about his own facial expressions, his own emotional state is reflected, which he can use to become more aware of himself. This is only possible through a specific marking in the caregiver's expressions of emotion; the marking indicates that the affect expressed by the parents applies to the child himself. The mechanism of this marking is not exactly deciphered and represents one of those still to be solved secrets of the interpersonal interaction. Due to the mirroring of the affect and the increasing awareness of the emotional state, the child can develop secondary control structures that positively regulate the states of affect in the child. The active modification of emotions in the interaction with caregivers is referred to as affect attunement [143]. Impairments in emotional dialogue have an impact on the child's affect regulation, so caregivers—if they react insensitively to the child and interrupt intentions to act, or respond to child signals through unpredictable behavior—can negatively shape affect regulation in the child. Empirical studies on mother-child communication have provided convincing evidence of this [33].

All forms of abuse and neglect have a significant impact on emotional dialogue and the development of emotional structures in the child. Child protection is and remains a fundamental challenge for child and adolescent psychiatry. The development of children with impaired parent-child relationships is an important open area of research [145].

Another interactive mechanism has a significant impact on affect regulation and the development of self-control in the child: it is called "social referencing" [146]. Social referencing as a form of reinsurance refers to the tendency of the toddler to look at the mother when confronted with interesting or unsettling objects and to adapt his own reactions to her facial expression and voice. If the mother communicates an anxiety affect, the child itself can show an anxious reaction, but if she smiles reassuringly, the child can continue to show curiosity. Such social referencing processes can be used to communicate affective evaluations and share them between the caregiver and the child. In this way, the child's emotional reactivity can be influenced favorably. It is not only exposed to an unsettling environment, but can constitute meanings in dialogue with the caregiver. Such social referencing also serves not only for early affective exchange, but also for the development of regulatory structures. In interaction with his caregivers, the child learns to find orientation, avoid stress and discover meaningfulness in unclear situations [147].

Emotional regulation problems are fundamentally involved in the development of psychopathological symptoms. The roots of such regulatory disorders not only extend to the area of genetic and epigenetic regulatory mechanisms [148], they also point to the importance of the early interaction processes between caregivers and children. The development of adolescent risk behaviors and psychopathological symptoms cannot be understood without the psychosocial context.

3.2.5 Stress and Trauma

Affects generate circumscribed activity patterns of the brain in a certain period of time, which are also called "state of mind" [149]. Such emotional states not only determine perception processes, but any evaluation of external and internal stimuli. Anyone who anxiously scans the area for dangers will be more likely to see signs of potential threats than someone who looks forward to a re-encounter. Certain emotional states also allow only very specific access to memory content: Affects thus (according to [150]) have a lock function for memory content [151]. It is quite clear that in emotional states of joy, grief or anger the perceptual functions and assessments of the environmental conditions—indeed the entire behavioral repertoire—can assume different intensities and qualities. States of Mind coordinate the adaptation activities of the individual. If emotional states rather indicate a low to medium degree of activation, we speak of an affective normal situation, in which the cognitive readiness is optimally available—we also speak of the state of prudence [129]. However, the situation changes as the level of activation continues to increase, eventually leading to affective pressure. Flared up affective turbulence can take on the character of exceptional states (e.g. tantrums or states of profound dismay). In these states, perceptions, ideas and basic attitudes are so narrowed that the entire world view can be "tinted" [152]. In such affective exceptional states, there is massive pressure to act, which is also referred to as an affective alarm reaction. According to Perry et al. [153], affective alarm reactions reveal two components [154]. The *overexcitation continuum* is compared with the *dissociation continuum*.

In dangerous situations a state of overexcitation ("overexcitation continuum") may occur, in which attack or withdrawal reactions are initiated. We speak of the so-called "fight-flight dichotomy". The world is squeezed into a black-and-white scheme, and the decision to "fight or flight" has to be made [155]. As an expression of regulatory processes in the context of the stress situation, there is increased sympathetic activity of the autonomous nervous system and an activation of the adrenal cortex system (HPA-axis stimulation inducing an increase of corticoid hormone levels in blood). The noradrenaline system also plays a role in this alarm response and noradrenaline rises. Attack decisions are prepared by anger affects, a high level of excitement and the positive assessment of one's own power of action lead to attack behavior in social and territorial disputes [155]. In contrast, the escape behavior is initiated by fear/anxiety affects. This inclination corresponds to a high level of excitement, which goes hand in hand with the certainty of a lack of power to act and tendencies to avoid. However, fear can also turn into aggressiveness, especially if it triggers traumatic experiences and an emergency appears inescapable—the phenomenon of courage in despair [156].

Affective alarm reactions can also be compensated for by interpersonal, affective co-regulation. With affective attunement and social referencing processes with important caregivers, the child can better cope with extraordinary stressful situations. The attachment context [157] and the emotional dialogue therefore play a fundamental role in affective regulation in alarm situations.

If the child is not protected by helping caregivers in the attachment context, the child remains exposed to the escape or attack dichotomy (fight-flight), but if escape or attack are not possible under the conditions of an alarm reaction, because both options are not permitted—but the danger remains present, it happens to a further escalation level of the alarm status. The increasing irritation leads to a process of despair. If it is not possible to recruit caregivers who jump to avert danger and the child finds no social echo or resonance in the environment—because, for example, the caregiver himself is the cause of the alarm reaction!—the child remains exposed to its escalating affective response [155]. The regulatory mechanism of the affective alarm reaction that is now starting is called the "dissociation continuum". This alarm reaction corresponds to surrender in the animal kingdom, there is a freezing reaction and inner distance from the danger, which can also be compared to a "bird ostrich behavior". In addition to the sympathetic, the parasympathetic nervous system is also activated, blood pressure and heart rate can drop despite increased adrenaline levels. Mesolimbic-mesocortical-dopaminergic systems and the opioid system are also involved in the dissociation reaction [155]. The reaction allows an unbearable moment of danger to be switched off or supposedly undone, so there is inner distancing. In the persistent presence of danger, the individual pretends that there is no danger at all. The alienation to self and environment is the consequence. Cognitive processing is interrupted. However, in this way, an unbearable situation can be survived by dissociative reactions. In the longer term, however, dissociative reactions can have unfavorable developmental effects on the child's affect regulation if they are repeated. We assume that all alarm reactions that cannot be mitigated in the interaction with caregivers overwhelm the child's affect system and thus give rise to different psychopathological symptoms if they occur repeatedly [155].

Events that directly endanger not only the health and integrity of the body, but even life itself in the child, trigger affective alarm situations. These burdens are all the greater when the child cannot find a way out and parental caregivers are not available for reassurance. In this case, events can trigger psychological trauma through affective alarm reactions [155]. Shonkoff et al. [158] speak of "toxic stress" in contrast to "positive stress", which is only of short duration and medium intensity and can be ended by the availability of caregivers. Sensitive adults can help the child cope with the stressful event. In contrast, toxic stress lays the foundation for lifelong physical and psychological impairments (see below Sect. 3.3 and [158]).

Single event-like trauma, such as we find in natural disasters and accidents or in victims of acts of terrorism, is called type 1 trauma, whereas chronic overwhelming experiences, which are characterized by emotional abuse, sexual abuse and cumulative traumatization in a social context of neglect are called type 2 trauma [159]. Even single events such as the loss of a parent in early childhood can ultimately have process-effective consequences. Traumas are usually characterized by the confluence of the affective alarm response and the dissociative continuum. This can lead to disintegration of psychological functions, so that self-reflection is changed [155]. Dissociative mechanisms can subsequently have an unfavorable effect on the development of the child's personality, especially if children suffer from multiple re-victimizations and re-traumatizations in the sense of a repetition tendency [155]. Finally, unfavorable development conditions and severe communication disorders with the important caregivers can lead to the development of adolescent borderline syndromes or the development of somatization and dissociative disorders. Transgenerational traumas are currently being considered [160, 161]. Parental abuse experiences can be a risk factor for children's development. The issue was raised, that parents who were abused in their own childhood have a tendency to abuse their children themselves or watch such abuse by others without intervening. In addition, the symptoms of an abuse trauma appear to inhibit the ability to create a family environment that is protective for the child and to respond to the child's needs with appropriate sensitivity [155]. Mothers with abuse experiences show changes in emotional availability in terms of intrusive behavioral patterns [162]. Disorders of mother-child bonding as a result of experiences of abuse by the mother are also reported [163].

Infants cannot predict the caregiver's behavior in mothers who are not sensitive enough. As a result, the infants express their attachment needs in unsettling situations in an exaggerated and dramatic way to be noticed at all. In these situations, the infant's attachment system is chronically activated, whereby in stressful situations curiosity and desire to explore are reduced in favor of excessive attachment behavior. In other children, their signals are severely restricted according to proximity and contact so that they do not have to expose themselves to the rejecting or impulsive behavior of the mother [164]. In all of these cases of parent-child interaction disorder, we have to focus on this insecure or disorganized attachment organization.

3.3   Adverse Childhood Experiences (ACE's)

Since the years when Felitti [165] published his paper on the long-term consequences of incest, rape, and molestation, evidence has grown that adverse childhood experiences exert a profound influence on adult health [158, 166]. See Table 3.1.

Adverse childhood experiences do not only affect psychological well-being and foster risk behaviors, but they also play an important role on the physical condition in adulthood. The risk factors in the classical adverse childhood experiences-study [168] included multiple stressors like child abuse or neglect, parental substance abuse and maternal depression. The consequences are disruptions of brain circuitry and other organ changes or metabolic systems dysfunctions. Such dysregulations may contribute as precursors of later impairments in health status. Not only the stress regulation systems may be impaired but individuals are prone to greater risk for a variety of chronic diseases in the adult years. Unhealthy life-styles and adolescent risk-taking are strongly associated with early adverse experiences [158]. However, toxic stress may also directly cause alterations in immune function like exaggerated inflammatory markers which themselves are related to poor health outcomes as diverse as cardiovascular disease, viral hepatitis, liver cancer, asthma, chronic obstructive pulmonary disease, autoimmune disease, and poor dental health [158].

Thus, adverse childhood experiences exhibit their detrimental effects in two directions: they are not only risk factors for direct somatic disruptions with lifelong consequences, they also obviously trigger later risk behaviors in adolescents and young adults! In spite of these data, the influence of environmental parameters on risk behavior and psychopathology is still underestimated and neglected in favor of genetic parameters or inborn brain dysfunctions.

Table 3.1 Long term consequences of child abuse (odds ratios of associations) [167]

	Physical abuse	Emotional abuse	Neglect
Depressive disorders	1.54	3.06	2.11
Suicide attempts	3.4	3.37	1.95
Drug use	1.92	1.41	1.36
Risky sexual behavior	1.78	1.75	1.57

3.4   The Problem of Emotion Regulation

Since emotions represent an archaic wisdom of adaptation and survival [169], they provide the human being with time-tested responses to recurrent adaptive problems [170]. As an arousal-system, emotions create urgency to act and regulate. Just as has been stated emotions represent the integration of inborn affects into the field of cognitive information processing. Emotions represent affective-cognitive evaluations of the internal and external environments. Emotions are triggered when something important to us is at stake [170]. The spectrum of emotion induction reaches from virtually automatic fear or astonishment—like reactions to a snake—to indirect concerns about the words of another after considerable meaning analysis—like anger about an affront [140, 171, 172].

A manifold of definitions of emotion regulation exists in the literature, therefore the treatment of this topic is challenging. We use the most popular and broad definition of the Stanford group. Emotion regulation refers to the process by which emotions are influenced, as to quality, intensity and duration. Emotion regulation helps us navigate in the emotional field concerning experience and expression [170]. It should be noted, that individuals may increase, maintain or decrease negative and positive emotions. Emotion regulation consists of conscious activities, but includes also processes without conscious awareness [170]. The question is still in dispute as to how far we can actively direct and control our emotions, or how much emotions can also control our experiences and we are passively delivered to them.

Several emotion regulation strategies have been described and assessed by several groups. Antecedent-focused emotion regulation has been contrasted with response-focused strategies [170]. Antecedent-focused strategies include situation selection, situation modification, attentional deployment and cognitive change. Situation selection can be very effective, e.g. when avoidance is adopted. To avoid a situation may prevent the person from resulting emotions—however, avoidance exerts a detrimental negative effect on further development. The person cannot grow in a shell of avoidance. Situation modification and attentional deployment are more specific strategies to problem focused coping, the selection of one of the situational aspects allows harm reduction neglecting others for the moment. All these strategies manipulate our experience of the situation due to emotions and not due to necessary environmental demands. Important adjustment options may be overlooked because perception remains restricted. This can lead to disturbances in the environmental relationship and situational control. Modification and selection strategies carry the disadvantage of a loss of control. Cognitive changes try to restructure the situation in our mind in a way that it better fits our expectations and goals neglecting the relation to reality of possible emotional irritations. Reappraisal refers to the selecting which of the many possible meanings will be attached to one's own perception. Cognitive change may decrease the emotional response; however, it may also be used to magnify the response or even change the emotion itself [170]. "The personal meaning that is assigned to the situation is crucial because it powerfully influences which experiential, behavioral, and physiological response tendencies will be generated in that particular situation" ([170]: 283). The reality-character of such a personal meaning will be discussed later. Should we attribute wrong meanings to situations only to calm down our emotional response? Again, such a strategy will be associated with a loss of control over the environment.

Response-focused emotion regulation consists of response modulation and suppression. Response modulation refers to attempts to influence emotion expression and mitigate the response into a socially accepted form [170, 173]. In other definitions, each process of regulating emotions aims to use cheap and socially appropriate behavioral strategies and that emotion regulation is adapted to the environment. Strictly speaking, this means that even the solving of a situational problem is dedicated to the emotion regulation including the aspect of situational adaptation [174]. An exaggerated definition of emotion regulation, which also includes all forms of problem solving and situational adaptation, makes every human action to be part of emotion regulation. In the narrower sense, the term should be limited to those actions and strategies that are intended to reduce emotional pressure without referring to environmental reality (see below).

Individuals seem to regulate their emotions in a wide variety of ways. John and Gross [173] focused on reappraisal (cognitive change of meaning) and suppression (change of situational emotion expression) in a study to find out, which way of regulation may be healthier than the other. Reappraisal was related to greater expression of positive emotions in self-reported and peer-reported measures. Reappraisal was also related to less negative-emotion experiences. Individuals frequently using suppression techniques experienced fewer positive emotions. Suppression could not diminish momentary negative emotion experience. In everyday life, suppression strategies may serve to increase negative affect instead (with its link to unauthenticity as the authors argue). No data could be collected on the relation to the subject's reality, whether the behavior of the situation was appropriate or not, because the study design did not take this aspect into account.

Emotion regulation itself is a developmental phenomenon. Emotion regulation starts as a co-regulation with caregivers as has been shown with the emotional dialogue. Parents thereby influence the development of emotional regulation in a dyadic process. Emotion regulation is a key component of emotional intelligence. The recognition and regulation of emotions in self and others has an important impact on interactions with peers in adolescents. Parent's emotion regulation as a model and the parent-child interactions shape emotional skills of the children and may influence the development of the children's regulatory (neuro)circuitry [175]. Emotion regulation skills develop substantially across adolescence [176]. Self-report studies robustly identified associations between emotion dysregulation and adolescent anxiety and depression. However, such dysfunctionalities may specifically be successfully addressed by psychological interventions focusing on improvement of emotion regulation [177].

The subject of emotion regulation has become ubiquitous in clinics and research. The hope is nurtured that an understanding of the regulatory mechanisms could lead to a new understanding of the pathogenesis of a large number of mental disorders. Therapy opportunities are also promised. However, do psychiatric problems and risk behaviors really result from a problem of emotion regulation in adolescents?

Are such primary defects leading up to psychopathology? Or could it be that everything is the other way around? Maybe we are all chasing a phantom here and maybe we should take a different view on the affects and emotions.

Affects and the resulting expressions and experiences of emotions are signs of (indicators of an urgency to change for) a discrepancy between a target value and a currently experienced state of the individual. Urgency has been signaled, there is pressure to act. The current situation is unsustainable and unbearable. As already mentioned definitions of emotion regulation include measures to repress tensions or change meanings without changing the situation on one side of the spectrum up to the point where the problem is solved to relieve the emotional pressure on the other end of the spectrum—which corresponds to the entire behavioral repertoire being subordinated to the term emotion regulation. Such over-inclusive definitions always apply, but do not seem helpful empirically. Because solving the problem is different from a suppression or denial strategy. We should restrict the definition of emotion regulation to processes actively involved to change emotion without changing the environmental demands.

It is probably overemphasized that the disruption of regulatory processes in the affective system consists of a primary regulatory disorder with an organic origin in most cases. The leading idea states, that a genetically determined dysfunction, or an age-related temporary restriction of somatic regulatory processes forms the basis of vulnerability, leading to emotional overreactions and affectively triggered psychopathological symptoms. However, this may not be true in most cases! In many cases, former experiences have led to the conclusion that the environment can be dangerous and that other people may be intrusive. Therefore, reactions to other people may be overwhelming and excessive. The emotional turmoil then is a realistic answer to environmental stress although it seems pathological from a clinical point of view. Excessive emotional reactions should not only be suppressed or prone to a reappraisal ("everything is not that bad") but the therapist should know that some adolescents react as they do, because for them it is harm avoidant, beneficial, and helpful in their eyes. The patient's evaluation of the environment should be the focus of interventions, not the intensity of the emotional expression!

Only in those rare cases, if persisting toxic stress may have distorted regulatory neuro-circuits (the brain reflects the past experience in neural plasticity), and dysfunctional psychic structure elements have been developed with overwhelming emotional reactions due to traumatic experience an additional help in applying regulatory strategies may seem fruitful.

Considering "Perceptual Control Theory" (see Chap. 8), the focus of the evaluation of the environment can be operationalized. Risk behavior may be due to an excessive emotional arousal as a signal for an urgent need to change one's situation. Self-worth and identity feelings have to be stabilized while the individual is dealing with an overwhelming environment. Risk behaviors may be an attempt to regulate the discrepancy between one's goals and the actual environmental necessities or demands. What is the goal of our interventions as therapists? Successful interventions do not primarily deal with emotion regulation, but rather with an optimization of the adaptation, which then allows the affect to subside.

Chapter 4
Contextual Development

4.1 How Do Risk Behaviors and Psychopathological Symptoms Develop?

Developmental psychopathology has broadened our interdisciplinary view of mental disorders in the last decades of the twentieth century and has been established to this day through its modeling of functional psychopathology—especially in child and adolescent psychiatry and psychotherapy. The basic idea of functional psychopathology is the adaptive value of psychopathological symptoms. Symptoms are not only an expression of disturbed brain functions—as often postulated by a nosology-oriented psychiatry—but represent the best possible adaptation of an individual in a particular time window, which can be achieved due to the resource situation. It is therefore necessary to consider environmental conditions and adaptation options together, because in this case, the symptom would not be a sign of disease per se, but the best solution to the discrepancy between requirements and resources.

The development of and therapeutic approach towards adolescent risk behaviors are presented differently in the light of developmental psychology and developmental neurobiology. They may be integrated into a "control loop context" from the point of view of adaptation and coping. The idea of functional properties of even pathological behaviors should not only change the view of genesis, epidemiology, and the type and expression of symptoms, but also enable new formulations for diagnostics, therapy, rehabilitation and prevention [57]. The focus is therefore on the influences of normal development on the presentation of psychopathological symptoms in different ages, just as the influence of psychopathological symptoms on normal development in the life cycle is viewed in the opposite sense. Due to different somatic, social, cognitive, and emotional conditions, children—and adults—have different resources in different phases of life to respond to mental shocks, traumas, and/or psychological crises in the struggle for adaptation to the environment. Mental disturbances reflect the expressions of a discrepancy between

F. Resch, P. Parzer, *Adolescent Risk Behavior and Self-Regulation*,
https://doi.org/10.1007/978-3-030-69955-0_4

requirements for adaptation and coping resources. Therapeutic processes never lead back to a—virtual—starting point in the sense of "healing", the direction of the developmental process can only be changed after a disruption/distortion and the process may hopefully run more favorably in the aftermath (see Chap. 3).

In this respect, symptoms and risk behaviors do not merely represent a brain disturbance but reflect a disturbance in the adaptation process of the individual in a given environment! The focus must be directed from the isolated individual towards the individual-environmental context in the sense of an eco-system in a certain time-frame. No static causality models can explain what is happening, but dynamic control loop models are needed. The Perceptual Control Theory offers an important explanatory model and is described in Chap. 8.

As a rule, the development of risk behaviors and psychopathological symptoms goes through several stages that can be distinguished from one another [54, 57, 129]:

Phase 1 is characterized by a biographically developed disposition: genetic liabilities (e.g. for mood disorders), childhood somatic developmental influences (e.g. malnutrition or epilepsy) and psychosocial developmental influences (e.g. relationship and educational factors when interacting with important caregivers) form the matrix of a disposition in various combinations. The dispositional resources or vulnerabilities represent the integral result of individual and interactional risk factors, protective factors and traumatic influences that affected the individual in childhood. One can also call this disposition psychic structure (see Chap. 6).

With this complex disposition, the individual enters the phase of adolescence and has to face new adaptation demands of age-specific development tasks and fateful life events (e.g. traumas and/or everyday adversities) at a certain point in age—this is the beginning of *phase 2*. In this area of challenges, the adolescent's adaptability is put to the test. Disposition-related adjustment turbulences and problems, which reflect a mismatch between coping options and challenges, ultimately cause emotional control problems as "irritations" according to the amount of problems [54]. These irritations manifest themselves as emotional understeer, a lack of control ("acting out" or "impulsive behavior") or emotional oversteer and over-control (behavioral inhibition, compulsiveness).

Phase 3 begins with a crisis-like adjustment problem if problems do not appear to be solvable and the adolescents come under massive pressure. Various attempts of coping have not led to success and the adolescents need self-repair mechanisms to withstand their own emotional pressure. Risk behaviors now set accents, which serve to maintain self-esteem and identity. Combat drinking, drug abuse, addictive internet consumption or other risk behaviors can shape the clinical picture. In addition, subclinical affective symptoms, exhaustion, sleep disorders or lack of motivation can be identified. This phase may be equally characterized by reluctance to personal contact, irritability, and tendencies to withdraw. Adolescents are still responsive to important others in their adaptation efforts and can still manage to cope with new situations. However, the degrees of freedom in their options for action are already limited [57].

If the mismatch to a family or non-family problem persists, a trauma cannot be dealt with, a developmental task cannot be solved, *phase 4* now occurs. Dispositional

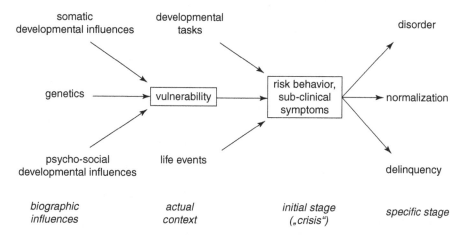

Fig. 4.1 Possible developmental pathways to disorder

vulnerability, or persistent risk behaviors can cause psychopathological symptoms in some adolescents that already allow a nosologically exact definition. In addition to the mental disorder, risk behaviors—such as substance abuse, delinquency, aggressiveness or self-harm—can complicate the clinical picture, or comorbidities of different nosological syndromes can cause more complex mental disorders. While phase 3 is still to be understood as a subclinical stage, phase 4 achieves a clinically significant condition requiring therapy.

Psychiatric disturbances do not appear all at once, but develop over preliminary stages and subclinical phases. Risk behaviors should be assessed as an expression of overwhelmed attempts by the adolescent to adapt to their environment. They are of great importance to the adolescent's self. In the further course, if the adjustment crisis does not come to an end, however, they pave the way for the occurrence of mental disorders. Risk behaviors can also create complex mental problems together with psychopathological features (see Fig. 4.1).

Chapter 5
The Biopsychosocial Model and Behavioral Presentation

The developmental model that underlies a functional analysis of symptoms in developmental psychopathology is the interactionist development theory [178]. Influences of nature and culture, civilization norms, and expectations of caregivers as well as natural environmental conditions are development incentives and represent developmental tasks that must be mastered by the individual. The peculiarity of the interactionist theory is that it gives the individual an active role in shaping his environment and does not degrade it to the passive place of action of different development influences.

Functional psychopathology is based on a homeostatic concept of adaptation. Man—as a multidimensional being—is in interaction with his environment. A systemic approach is necessary to understand this interrelation. Seen in this way, humans themselves are complex systems that work by integrating multiple subsystems, and this system interacts with a multidimensional complex environment. The individual-environment interaction itself can again be viewed as a meta-system. A deepening of the systems theory perspective can be done at [179–181].

The individual strives for the greatest possible degree of psychological homeostasis as part of his adaptation efforts. It is important to note that individuals are not looking for a state of lack of tension or rest, but a state of optimal stimulation between under-stimulation and irritation [134]. Even newborns are actively challenged by the environment. If the adaptation needs prove to be too high, they lead to emotional turbulence. In this context, the importance of individual goals cannot be overestimated. The goal as a target idea has a pulling effect on all reactions and actions of the individual in dealing with the environment. Each goal itself is in turn complex and contains hierarchically integrated sub-goals. This creates a directionality that characterizes all human activities and actions, each sub-action pursues a sub-goal and integrates experiences in the field of forces of the present [134]. The transformed past, which is laid down in structural features of the self (Chap. 6), updates itself in the wake of a draft for the future, the self is guided by its goals, whereby the continuous interaction between the self and the environment can also

F. Resch, P. Parzer, *Adolescent Risk Behavior and Self-Regulation*, https://doi.org/10.1007/978-3-030-69955-0_5

appear to be a logical consequence of what has been done so far (the behavior is the result of former social conditions)—this double view interprets the same action based on the past as it recognizes behavior as a future-oriented necessary step towards a goal (just pursuing a purpose).

We rarely have to deal with one-dimensional causal chains in the context of human action. Because a behavioral answer as a logical consequence of the previous one, is usually not mandatory in its singularity, but there are several possibilities of behavioral answers [134]. Previous behaviors and risks always leave room for maneuvers in the context of the consequences. Whether and in what form the individual benefits from such a current range of behavior, which the disposition of development and the situational circumstances allow, how the individual acts in this range depends on the individual target variables—the goals. The action will take a nuanced different form, depending on whether the inner goal is to maximize feelings of pleasure, avoid discomfort or actions in the service of self-development or the fulfillment of a need for commitment. Clinical explorations should track down such "guidelines" in the human biography and make internal goals recognizable. (This will be discussed in more detail in Chap. 9).

However, psychopathological models that focus on both risk behaviors and psychotherapy cannot avoid focusing on a functional view of psychopathological phenomena and thus continuing an old tradition of psychotherapy, starting with Freud's notions [182] and in the early behavioral therapy followed by Skinner [183]. Both opened up a new way of understanding for the psychopathological phenomena [57]. Functional psychopathology makes it clear that symptoms not only mean deficits, but can also be useful and serve goals in the context of life.

The simple classic causality models of a genetic, brain-organic or experience-reactive derivation of current symptoms—with their "either-or" character—have been abandoned in favor of more complex notions of vulnerability [184]. A number of empirical studies attempt to find interactions between genetic or neurobiological factors and experience-reactive variables that make certain individuals more sensitive or more resilient to negative environmental constellations and traumatic situations [185–188]. Groundbreaking discoveries in these areas (summary by [189]) are always countered by sobering failed attempts to replicate important findings [190]. But even these most complex causal models cannot avoid relating current states of suffering primarily to the past and should be supplemented by those aspects that concern the present and the future: from a functional perspective of the psychopathological symptoms, the question of the inner motives is also asked. The question is less about what a symptom is derived from, but more about what purposes and future-oriented goals a symptom can serve. Such considerations are not primarily directed against the causal derivation, but rather should supplement it with new considerations and views [57].

If one wants to focus on risk behavior, one cannot avoid the common bio-psycho-social model (see Chap. 2). The bio-psycho-social model superficially meets these needs for a multi-dimensional, integrative perspective. However, a closer look reveals that the bio-psycho-social model, both in biological and in social and psychological areas, is formulated in different languages [62]:

The biosphere is spelled out in the language of the natural sciences, the newer research approaches have very differentiated multilevel conceptions on the somatic level, in the context of which correlative relationships to the psychological phenomena are established, whereby these are mostly implicitly interpreted causally—the psychological processes follow the somatic correlates: first comes the soma—from this follows the psyche. The steps from the somatic prerequisites to the psychological processes remain rudimentary and woodcut-like [62]. The causal relationships often are deduced from the correlations and considered—which is actually not legitimate. Couldn't the somatic conditions simply depict mental processes and actually follow them instead of always leading them?

The social field is also subject to the empirical method of investigation and is open to the scientific vocabulary. Attachment and social structures, discursive rules and codes of conduct are clarified that define and shape the child's (and adult's) freedom of behavior and development. Causal relationships, which also clearly claim validity in individual cases, do not shape the picture. Rather, social developmental influences remain at the level of "increased probability", as we know it from all risk research [62].

The psychic level in the bio-psycho-social model has a Janus-headed double structure. It is the affective-cognitive activity of the subject that is of great importance in the external perception of itself and others as well as in the self-reflection of the internal perception. The subjective side of man is no longer the "black box", which is determined from the outside in its control functions. The inside perspective—or first-person perspective—is not to be directly connected to the outside perspective—or third person perspective. There is no epistemological bridge, there are no explicative transitions between the two [191]. The boundary between inside and outside cannot be resolved epistemologically [62]. Nevertheless, as therapists, we have to operate repeatedly at this border and mediate between different levels of the bio-psycho-social model in order to remain able to act.

The recognition of man as a subjective being must not be sacrificed to the preponderance of neurobiological explanatory models [192], even if there are no continuous logical steps between the subject perspective and the object perspective. Our soul is not an epiphenomenon of neuronal processes, the language of "neuronal noise" cannot grasp the utterances of the subject! Each domain of the bio-psycho-social model has its own traditions and different language usage. A multi-level model of the human psyche is therefore more similar to a multi-language model in the Wittgenstein sense of "language games" [193]. Anyone who moves in the bio-psycho-social model must repeatedly oscillate between different starting points, systems of thought and forms of observation and also cross scientific language boundaries [63]. On the other hand, if you only stay in one language (e.g. the language of the natural sciences), you have a too narrow view of the interrelations and therefore only have limited ability to act from a therapeutic point of view. We have repeatedly demanded that there be respect and tolerance between different perspectives of the person in order to create a climate of reciprocity. Because if any form of therapeutic help is "help for self-help", then the human perspective cannot be limited to a machine model of neuronal functions [194].

The biological processes follow the causality of natural processes and can be spelled out mathematically. Social relationships, risk factors and milieu conditions are often formulated in the domain of epidemiology and covered by the laws of statistics. Depending on the question, the psychological responsibilities, emotions, thoughts and behavior are measured scientifically and empirically (objectifying) and then interpreted in the humanities (subject-oriented) or they are the result of primarily introspective procedures and derived from self-reports (narratives or questionnaires). Psychological interpretations often represent complex assessments that allow thoughts and behavior to be poured into communicative forms in dialogical situations. This corresponds to the clinical context.

However, in different clinical approaches, the different viewing levels are linked with one another, the question of when and at what point in time an intervention should be applied often remains open in everyday clinical practice. The question is: when do I use which verbal intervention, when do I give a medication, how do I interpret therapy success, at which level of the bio-psycho-social model is therapy successful? What are the reasons for which treatment failure is attributed to which consideration? How should we interpret interventions at multiple levels that take place simultaneously (such as psychotherapy and pharmacotherapy)? Where does what work when? Could there possibly also be opposing therapeutic effects?

Our knowledge and interventions as psychotherapists combine different methods of cognition in the natural and social sciences with a hermeneutic point of view [63]. Since there is no closed meta-theory that allows meta-evaluations within the individual domains of the bio-psycho-social model, the therapist's decisions are based on his own ability to simultaneously interpret different fields of knowledge and integrate them for a professional performance. What makes one or the other aspect in the bio-psycho-social model come to the fore? On closer inspection, it is probably nothing but the personal clinical experience that is effective in a controlled and reflective manner. The self-reflective weighting and assessment of different findings is therefore not solely based on a theory, but on a clinical assessment that allows our therapeutic decisions to be made on a value-oriented basis [63]. From a theoretical perspective, this must leave us unsatisfied. How can the practical relevance of the therapist's decision be substantiated, settled and improved? It seems that the context for different therapeutic decisions in the biological, biographical or social area is a highly individual, experience-dependent, almost private intentional subjective space [63]. The evaluation of clinical phenomena always requires values, which have to be reflected. This cannot be provided by natural science knowledge proof alone. Evidence without experience is nothing.

So far, the bio-psycho-social model appears to be only slatternly soldered at the different viewing and therapy levels [63]. There is no convincing meta-language that allows the bio-psycho-social model to be formulated unanimously. However, an approach that deals with the phenomenon of the functionality of symptoms in control loops could also emphasize a common point of view for different viewing levels. The functional consideration of psychopathological phenomena can formulate an aspect in the context of the bio-psycho-social model in one language—namely that of system theory—in the control loop concept. This idea of the control loop will therefore be discussed later (see Chap. 8).

Even if some authors [195] made the demand to implement increasingly disorder-specific and nosologically modularized psychotherapeutic interventions, this has to be critically examined in adolescents for several reasons. There are arguments in favor of the psychotherapeutic indication for psychotherapy that seriously question the concept of nosology-specificity.

Especially in adolescents risk behaviors [57], but also in psychotherapeutic intervention research in general [196], the problem of comorbidity is a major obstacle to nosology-specificity. It has been shown repeatedly that adolescents generally do not have one clearly defined mental disorder, but also present an abundance of comorbid syndromes that cannot be neglected therapeutically [197]. In addition, there are always individual subliminal psychological symptom constellations that do not meet a diagnostic category, but can be grasped in a dimensional way as subjective impairment. Bastine [196] concludes in his considerations that in psychotherapeutic practice, the multiple, often interrelated mental disorders place great demands on the practicing psychotherapists, which are simply not manageable with disorder-specific concepts and manuals.

In addition, symptoms and behaviors can escalate in young people depending on the situation, for example in the home environment or in the school context; whereby these build-ups go hand in hand with conflicts typical of young people and can give rise to current emotional turbulence and problematic risk behavior due to the different reactions of the adults. Developmental tasks, such as searching for identity or regulating self-esteem, also contribute to the overall symptom picture of adolescents; depersonalization phenomena can then complicate the symptom picture (for a more detailed explanation of this topic, see [57]). Especially in adolescents, a current problem pressure, existential questions ("What do I actually live for"), questions of origin (e.g. with adopted or foster children), disappointments in love relationships, sexual fears or concerns about the future lead to a further escalation of existing symptoms that then bring new risks through additional risk behaviors such as self-harm or substance abuse. Vital impairments and sleep disorders are then present, without the diagnostic category of depression being able to be crystallized in full screen [57]. All of these considerations contribute to the fact that from a psychotherapeutic point of view, a strictly nosology-oriented approach does not appear to make sense for the psychotherapy of adolescents [194]. It is the risk behavior that matters. The voluntary life-styles following the inner goals of young people do form the adolescent's reality.

Chapter 6
Psychic Structure, Personality and Psychodynamics

Psychotherapy in adolescents can not only focus on discontinuing and alleviating psychopathological symptoms, but should also consider the cognitive-emotional resources of the person, give importance to affect regulation and life issues, and focus on internal conflicts and interactional problem issues. The psychic structure and the development of the self-concept are of central importance. The role of memory cannot be neglected when considering conscious and unconscious processes. The development of "mentalization" [34] also plays an important role in the development of psychological structures.

From a psychodynamic point of view, it therefore makes sense not only to consider the meanings of the development context, but also to grasp the relationship patterns, the psychic structure, possible persistent conflicts and subjective dimensions of the treatment motivation in a special way [47].

While the concept of the psychic structure has a high level of intuitive evidence, when attempting exact definitions, it largely eludes a conceptual version. Everything we call structure represents a static element in the dynamics of the development process. The structure is what remains, it represents the crystallization of the current, vital memories that remain of the life process as experiences and are made available to the next step in life. The psychic structure is connected with memory as well as with temperament, perceptual characteristics, and behavioral style [198]. Two aspects of the term structure should be emphasized:

- The psychic structure shows a direct connection to areas of memory and experience. The current is recorded and transformed into enduring forms of knowledge.
- The second aspect of psychic structure concerns the renewal, i.e. the repeated provision of what is already known, the utilization of experience in the context of the adaptation process [141].

Psychic structures (the plural form seems more appropriate) serve as order categories of the psyche and organizers of life processes both vital to the survival of the individual itself and in the interpersonal communication. Psychic structures serve

F. Resch, P. Parzer, *Adolescent Risk Behavior and Self-Regulation*, https://doi.org/10.1007/978-3-030-69955-0_6

both self-regulation and affect control, as well as the refinement of the perception processes of self and others. The ability to establish appropriate contacts and regulate proximity and distance also makes use of the repertoire of psychic structures as a communicative ability. Since all representative human stocks can be understood as layered, hierarchically organized control loops, which can be specifically effective in different adaptation processes, the term is used in its plural form: psychic structures (see Chap. 8).

6.1 The Self

The self-concept is also multi-layered and hierarchically organized. It consists of different modules of experience that are linked to each other in a high degree of complexity. Self-experience arises in the context of interpersonal experience [199]. According to Frank [200], the self as an experience results from an indissoluble, immediate acquaintance of the subject with itself—the self begins as an immediate self-assurance. Such spontaneous awareness as a living being and actor in adaptation processes is not conveyed objectively or conceptually, but seems to arise from an immediate experience from within. It is only in a second reflective step—i.e. self-reflective processes—that a physical, spatio-temporal determination of the person comes about [199]. Self-reflection can be understood as part of the perception and allows vital basic experiences of existence. If the subject has become an empirical object for itself, this leads to the phenomena of self-awareness and self-confidence (see Chap. 1).

In the further development of a structural model by Damon and Hart [201], we described the structural model of the self in detail in 2009 [199]. We referred to earlier considerations [129, 147]. This structural formulation of the self should be illustrated here:

A subjective self, which is conceptualized as an immediate instance of experience, is juxtaposed with a self-reflective, expanded, complex structure—the definitory self [202]. In the following, the model definitions for subjective and definitory self from Resch [199] are cited with minor modifications.

The subjective self or self as a subject can be understood as a structural control instance of the person. The subjective self is based on an implicit mental model, which develops as a decision-making body of action tendencies in the first year of life from the complexity of neural networks in the adaptation to the environment. Information processing, motivation and the preparation of actions are the central tasks. As an implicit mental model, the subjective self also contains unconscious parts of actual and earlier life experiences and unconscious decision criteria. It forms the basis of the person and corresponds to the reflective evidence of a thinking, feeling and acting human being. The subjective self is closely tied to affective processes and corresponds to an immediate, holistic, first-hand experience in the context of life [203]. The subjective self or self as a subject includes all aspects of self-awareness and self-evidence. As a schema, the subjective self is subject to changes in the context of development, as cognitive developmental steps of adopting perspectives and the increasing ability of self-reflection also change the type of self-awareness. The dimensions of self-determination as experiences of one's own will and personal control, the delimitation from other people and things as well as the uniformity and consistency across different emotional states characterize the subjective self, depending on the situation and over time. The self-reflective confirmation of the subjective self leads to a feeling of identity (see Chap. 1). It corresponds to the self-awareness of a holistic ego experience [199].

In contrast, the definitory self is seen as the result of a differentiated objectifying self-knowledge by self-reflection, which is fed from the autobiographical, episodic and semantic memory (see below in the text). The self becomes the starting point for an explicit self-examination and modeling. The definitory self thus represents the entirety of affective, cognitive information about the self. Perceptions about oneself, evaluations of one's own actions are processed, which lead in the interpersonal context beyond an immediate holistic ego experience. The self is fixed in the explicit memory as a definitory self and can be divided into four domains. We differentiate between [202]:

- A body-self, which represents all somatic attributes and emotional experiences in connection with the own body (body experiences). It encompasses all forms of training and self-optimization, reflections on size, strength and beauty, embellishment, adornment, body images and body feelings.
- An acting self, the representation of the active person, her/his skills, abilities and actuations; it encompasses all forms of active action on objects, problem solving and the effects on reality.
- A social self develops from experiences in an interactive context and is a result of experienced inter-subjectivity. Experience of attachment, social echo and communication with peers play an important role.
- An emotional or spiritual self (value self) finally is defined. It encompasses those emotionally borne basic experiences, values, structures of meaning and preferences, desires and fantasies, which form the basis of our philosophy of life. This spiritual self represents a source of experiences and activities that give creativity, depth and dignity to people [198].

The self has auto-regulatory skills. It knows multiple objectives, allows subject experiences, becomes active in self-regulatory processes and can be tangible in its reactions to the environment as well as in intentional efforts. It is ultimately realized through actions in a social context [199, 202].

Psychic structures develop as auto-regulatory building blocks in an interactive context. Psychic structures contain hierarchically layered experiences that serve to regulate interpersonal communication and one's own emotional tensions. According to the theory of William T. Powers [180, 204], psychological structures in cybernetic formulations can be understood as hierarchically ordered systems of control loops that control behavior as stratified hierarchies of meaning. Each control loop is based on its own goal, which represents its reference value. The theory of Powers here is a powerful model for affect-logical structures [150] and could play a fundamental role in the further development of the concept of the psychic structures in the future (see Chap. 8).

6.2 Memory

The psychic structure of the self naturally exists as a basic memory structure. All affect-logical experiences are closely tied to memory [199]. In a brief overview of different forms of memory, according to Squire [205] we can distinguish two groups of forms of memory [206]. The declarative memory is also referred to as the explicit memory, it can be contrasted with the non-declarative—or implicit—memory. Experiences are stored in the declarative memory, which can be explicitly recorded via working memory and saved in learning processes. Such memory contents can ultimately be called up and reproduced consciously. In contrast, the non-declarative memory contains experiences and action tendencies that implicitly—below the threshold of consciousness—control our behavior [199]. Since non-declarative memory has been made available to man from birth, it will be examined in more detail below [202, 206]:

- Priming effects identify horizons of meaning for images, faces and words and automatically create semantic links. This memory function creates "without conscious action"—important links of meaning that relate to events, objects and word content.
- Classic and operant conditioning processes can guide our behavior below the threshold of consciousness, without us gaining evidence about it.
- Habituation and sensitization processes influence our future behavior based on experiences without having to have self-reflective access. In the context of stress reactions, this memory mechanism can give rise to implicit readiness to react, which allows us to act in certain key moments in a certain way without being able to account for it. In this way, especially under traumatic conditions, willingness to act can be evoked with which no conscious memories of the trauma may have to be linked.
- Perception, action and thinking routines (such as driving a car or playing the piano) are procedural skills that are also stored in non-declarative memory. Through these routines, willingness to behave comes about, which allows routine actions to take place below the threshold of consciousness.

The non-declarative (implicit) memory influences our experience and behavior fundamentally. Emotional regulation and self-regulation are not only based on explicit memory experiences, but also on implicit structure-building memory mechanisms.

The declarative (or explicit) memory of experience only develops in the course of the first year of life and, with language development, reaches a new level of complexity in childhood [199]. It can be divided into an episodic and a semantic memory. In episodic memory (or experience memory), personal events and experiences are stored in a spatial-temporal reference system with affective, cognitive and self-related aspects. In contrast, the semantic memory is the archive in which old and newly learned facts as well as the overarching narrative world knowledge are collected. The declarative memory is in principle accessible to self-reflection [206].

It is therefore not surprising that early childhood experiences—which are primarily stored in implicit memory—are not immediately accessible to consciousness. It is only around the age of three that experiences can open themselves up to explicit access through memory functions in later ages. Early life experiences are simply procedurally anchored. Even if explicit storage and therefore later deliberate retrieval of memory contents are not yet possible in the early stages of memory development, tendencies to act in implicit memory are already significant for the development of the child's psychological structures. It remains to be seen whether such implicit readiness to act is also part of the substrate that can be assigned to the psychodynamic concept of the unconscious.

Even later in life, implicit and explicit memory storage does not always have to be coordinated as is usually the case. Especially under traumatic conditions, there can be a decoupling of implicit and explicit memory storage, since under extreme stress conditions the storage of experiences in working memory can be impaired in many ways. In such cases, it is conceivable that, under dramatic conditions, implicit memory storage can take place as a readiness to react to the corresponding triggers without a complete, explicit wealth of experience. The psychological structures that serve the self-regulation and control of communicative abilities are made up of both conscious and non-declarative building blocks [202].

6.3 Mentalization

The concept of mentalization has prevailed in the first decade of this millennium. Its most well-known representatives are Fonagy et al. [144, 207], who integrated psychoanalytic conceptions with attachment-theoretical considerations and empirical research results of the theory-of-mind concept into a whole. Mentalization can be seen as the ability to view other people and oneself as beings with mental, psychological states, whereby the person recognized as subject is capable of intersubjectivity, enables perspectives to be taken from one another's point of view and is ultimately capable of self-reflective knowledge [141]. The concept of mentalization appears to be closely related to reflective self-functions [34, 208]. The phenomenon of mentalization empowers people to foresee the behavior of others by using concepts of their own inner life for it and in this sense can presuppose an inner life of the other. Each subject develops a theory about what the other subject or one intends to do. The behavior of the other is seen as a result of subjective action and an understanding of the other subject is developed by dealing with what the other desires, hopes, longs for, rejects or maybe pretends [141]. Mentalization is more than just a cognitive achievement.

Mentalization begins as an unconscious and implicit memory function in infants. Mentalization also gives meaning to one's own experience and behavior. By the theory of mind, we mean the social perspective that begins to develop in the child at about the age of four. From this point on, the child is able to include the subjective constitution of others in his world of experience and action, and to explicitly differentiate the opinions and attitudes of others from his own point of view [141]. The mentalization process therefore begins from birth. Starting from a strictly interactional paradigm for intersubjectivity, Fuchs and De Jaegher [209] and Fuchs [210] criticize the mentalization concept as too cognitive and contrast it with another concept—the concept of enactive and embodied social cognition. In this theory, the understanding of other individuals arises, not only through mutual exchange of inner world references, but stems from an embodied social interaction, which can also be described as an intermediate body (see [199]). The basic emotional experiences that are given to both interaction partners in joint actions are mutually developed in the parent-child interaction. This creates implicit knowledge bases for relationships that predestine dealing with others. So (unconscious) behavioral prerequisites are created, how to share joy, attract attention, avoid rejection or re-establish lost contact [209]. Such primarily unconscious structural schemes of interpersonal interactions could be the prerequisite for conscious schemes of interpersonal relationships.

The two conceptions do not fundamentally contradict each other, since the mentalization concept also sees the root of the development of psychic structures in early implicit processes of experience.

The mentalization hypothesis assumes that the symbolic play in infancy (i.e. between 1.5 and 4 years) has the same status in the child that the interactional mirroring had in the first year of life. The focus is on two modalities in which thoughts and feelings are represented: the as-if mode ("pretend mode") and the mode of equivalence ("psychic equivalence mode") [211]. Both modalities can exist in parallel. The child can also oscillate between the two modalities. The two symbol modes are only integrated in the age group beyond 4 years after the social perspective taking has been adopted.

In the "pretend mode" the child can emphasize the contrast between play and seriousness. The psychic interior becomes a framework for imagination and scope for possibilities. In the symbolic game, representation possibilities are created to reflect one's own responsibility externally [30]. Feelings are effectively anchored in the characters [211]. Here too, affective modulation and reinsurance processes take place with the caregivers. Caregivers and children move in a space of possibilities, in a kind of representation of reality and not in reality itself [30]. The "as-if room" is a fantasy room, in which the child can walk about without danger. However, the child may quickly switch to the other mode of experiencing equivalents of reality with immediate concern, although they are still processed mentally and did not take place in reality.

In the "equivalence mode", the child experiences his thoughts as if they were real. In comparison to real experiences, ideas and fantasies of the "as-if" mode only have a remotely similar effect on the emotional system [30]. In contrast, experiences in the equivalence mode correspond fully to reality. The child is immersed in a "virtual reality". A case study may illustrate this: a child who playfully develops the idea in the bathtub that the escaping water could represent a dangerous vortex that could pull all objects down into the drain. This game is slowly becoming serious— the initially playful mode slips into the equivalence mode of being able to be grasped by this vortex itself and also being sucked into the drain [197]. The child starts to panic and considers his own imagination to be real. In this context too, how the caregiver deals with the child's experience is of particular importance [30]. Parents can take the child's feeling seriously and accept it, but at the same time distance themselves and make it clear that they are not experiencing the same thing. The parents thus join the child's perception, but keep a different perspective for the child [30]. In this way, parents can contribute to creating distance from the child's perspective in play [211]. So while the pretend mode characterizes the game as a fantasy mode, the equivalence mode takes effect in the sense of a virtual reality [197]. In the former case, the child can distance itself and refrain from it, it can also deal with emotionally stressful aspects in a distant and playful manner. In the equivalence mode, the child is involved and affected. This idea leads to irritation, imagination and reality mix. The game becomes serious.

6.4 Resources of the Self and the Structure of Symptoms

The psychic structures that develop—from a psychodynamic point of view—in childhood and adolescence assume that the child has a repertoire of willingness to act at any age, which the subject can use in interaction with the environment [141]. Psychic structures are understood to mean the functionality, flexibility, variability, continuity, and availability of action strategies and possibilities for processing experience; this enables a situation-appropriate coping with everyday life. Psychic structures are about psychological freedom for decision-making and the relationship of the self to its inner and outer objects [142]. The different dimensions of the psychic structures are described in detail in the operational diagnosis of psychodynamics in children and adolescents [47].

The better the psychic structures are developed, the better conflicts, adjustment turbulences or traumas can be processed internally [57]. Compensatory coping, problem-solving skills, and mature defense mechanisms for affect regulation are then available. The more serious structural impairments are to be diagnosed, the more the children or adolescents have to act out their conflicts, tensions, and psychological injuries in the outside world. Most psychopathological symptoms such as anxiety, depressive mood, obsessive-compulsive symptoms or different forms of risk behaviors appear to occur at different functional levels of the subject. From a structural point of view, these functional levels are of particular importance for the therapeutic indication. Depending on whether problems of self-control, disturbances of impulse management, impairments of self-awareness or disturbances of communication skills are linked with the symptoms, the intervention has to be done differentially. In a further development of a model by Kernberg [212], the symptom presentation is as follows [57, 202]:

- At *functional level one*—the reactive level—symptoms become tangible as current adaptation problems. There is a close connection to impairment due to developmental tasks or current dramatic events and threats. There are no previous limitations of psychological resources before the critical event happened. Regulatory and compensatory activities were only triggered by the current event. Basic functions of self-regulation and communication are also retained in the context of the symptoms.
- *Functional level two*—the conflict level—impresses with excessive reactions to triggers in the environment. These are over-reactions; the symptoms are exceptionally accentuated and appear inadequate in relation to the triggering situations. Previous traumas or persistent conflicts determine the symptoms, impairments of emotion regulation and hypersensitivity can be detected, the relationship to the emotional environment is complicated by rigid defense structures or compensatory behaviors and the communication processes in everyday life are thereby impaired (see also [57]).
- *Functional level three*—the narcissistic level—is defined by a profound impairment of self-regulation. The balance and maintenance of self-esteem appear to be permanently disturbed in central life contexts, therefore the clinical symptoms take place against a background of massive self-esteem problems, which not only cause excessive reactions, but also reflect fundamental fears of object loss. This means that the children and adolescents do not feel good enough to be able to keep important caregivers or peers stable in their lives. There is a fear of losing the other, of being despised, of having to hide a deep flaw, so that there are always new attempts at self-reflection. Negative self-attributions alternate with ideas of supposed size, idealizations and devaluations. There is greed for social echo, and at the same time, there are fears that this echo is unstable. There is an up and down between ideas of personal greatness and self-contempt, which complicates relationships with the outside world and communication with other people.
- *Functional level four*—the borderline level—reflects a profound disruption of self-integration. There are fears of self-loss, identity diffusion, as well as a disturbed self- and impulse regulation. The striking discontinuity in relationships still leaves a strong desire for a relationship. High levels of irritability go hand in hand with fear of disappointment. This can lead to chaotic forms of adaptation, there is a tendency to acting out, increased risk behaviors are noticeable. Dissociative symptoms can complicate self-reflection and give rise to experiences of self-alienation. A negative attitude towards the body and other fundamental distortions of the self-image become tangible. At this functional level, the individual shows himself disintegrated in his self and object representations. The self-image and the image of other people are not stable. However, the perceptive functions and the ability to control reality are not permanently switched off, but strongly affect-related and impaired in certain contexts.

- *Functional level five*—the psychotic level—is already characterized by a fragmentation of inner experience. Self-regulation and identity functions are fundamentally disrupted by profound impairments in information processing. Disturbances of perception and situational evaluation functions largely impair interpersonal interaction, so that a shared reality with other people cannot be established. There is a fundamental loneliness, a retreat into private worlds, which also seems permanently threatened. This creates severe suffering. Thought disorders and perception disorders can shape the clinical picture, at this level the basic "tool functions" of the psyche are already fundamentally impaired.

In childhood and adolescence, we typically find an oscillation that takes place between different levels of psychic structures in different contexts. This is important for an assessment in the sense of a psychodynamic diagnosis to record relatively persistent, structural readiness. Some psychopathological phenomena, such as anxiety and depression, can be clearly diagnosed at different structural levels of function with reference to the self-aspects. However, there are three disorder patterns that already have a strong structural relationship as nosological constructs [142]:

- Neurodevelopmental disorders, such as autism spectrum disorder, because in this case we generally find structural deformations up to functional levels four and five.
- In schizophrenic psychoses in the acute phase, we regularly find structural impairments up to functional level five.
- In adolescent borderline disorders there are complaints that can oscillate between level three and four and in individual contexts range up to functional level five (a more detailed discussion of these aspects can be found in [57]).

Risk behaviors in adolescents should be diagnosed using the functional levels of psychic structures in a way to differentiate between particular intervention strategies.

Chapter 7
Functional Contextualism and Goal Directed Behavior

If one has described the risk behaviors and psychopathological symptoms in detail, they need to be differentiated in their context (How do the patients suffer? In which way are the symptoms linked to each other and to the environment?). The next question that usually arises is the cause (Where do symptoms and behaviors come from? What are the causal conditions and antecedents of certain behaviors?). Many neuro-biological and socio-theoretical models attempt to describe clinical symptoms as a result of cerebral disorders and/or social constraints. The therapeutic steps based on these models are causally oriented and try to influence the causal conditions—e.g. a suspected lack of serotoninergic processes through medication or in the psycho-therapeutic field through the processing of biographical trauma—so that the clinical symptoms may decrease. However, these models assume that symptoms follow their causes almost reflexively or seem to be unconditionally driven by them. This is rarely the case and the therapeutic attempts may in many cases remain unsuccessful. We want to take a different view on symptoms and risk behaviors, which assumes that they always have an adaptive function and are embedded in their psychosocial contexts. Symptoms and behaviors always pursue inner goals and endowments, symptoms and behaviors aim at purposes (what for?).

The question of causality focuses on deriving behavior from preconditions; it presents behavior as a necessary consequence of such preconditions. Behavior is the conclusive result of these preconditions. From the point of view of the beholder, the symptoms of those affected are involuntary from a causal point of view, they happen to the patient, so to speak, they are not actively generated by them.

In most fields of action, however, the patients are given leeway which enables them to make a choice. The behavior can be controlled, applied and adapted to environmental conditions. Like every healthy person, the patient acts according to goals, he uses behavior to achieve goals. In this way, behaviors do not simply happen, they are created and actively started. Symptoms are not simply caused passively and happen by coercion, they are actively selected from a canon of possible behaviors. It seems important that action to achieve goals should not be equated with conscious

F. Resch, P. Parzer, *Adolescent Risk Behavior and Self-Regulation*,
https://doi.org/10.1007/978-3-030-69955-0_7

self-reflective action. Internal goals can also remain unconscious or be effective outside of attention. Many actions and behaviors take place permanently in a targeted manner in us, without exceeding our consciousness threshold. Anything that goes beyond the simple stimulus-reaction mechanism of reflex-like actions (referred to by the learning theories as "elicited behavior") can be described as active behavior (referred to in the learning theories as "emitted behavior"). Not every active behavior is consciously or self-reflectively chosen. Between the level of reflexes and self-conscious behavior there is a whole spectrum of goal directed behaviors with only a loose or non-existent reference to consciousness (see Chap. 8).

The causal view may normally serve an appropriate explanation for psychopathological symptoms (like hallucinations or depression). But for the same symptoms in other circumstances, the contextual functional view could appear more fruitful. No view has a single excluding truth, every view makes other phenomena recognizable.

In the experiences and behaviors that seem imposed on us primarily by causal processes—for example, epileptic convulsions, hallucinations or panic attacks—context variables may play a subordinate role in the initial development, but the context is very important in the maintenance, chronification or aggravation of such symptoms. However, where degrees of freedom for decisions exist from the beginning, where the person concerned has a choice to modify behavior or experience, where behavior is emitted in an environmentally-related way—in most human behavior—functional contextualism plays an outstanding role. Because in the design and perpetuation of behaviors, there are practically always degrees of freedom for the patient, that serve to achieve his inner goals. Knowing such goals opens up new scope for change when they are accessible to the conscious mind. We know that some purely causally oriented forms of therapy (e.g. pharmacological interventions directed towards dysfunctional processes of brain circuits) can fail due to behavioral control loops that perpetuate pathological behavior. Therapy resistance can develop in this way—not only due to pharmacokinetic variables or a lack of receptor sensitivity. If symptoms serve hidden motives they may be maintained to achieve these goals and thus counteract therapy. Regulated behavior always plays a role when context variables are important and a comparison with the environment takes place when internal goals guide our behavior as guidelines, motives and wishes.

A functional consideration of symptoms assumes that they always serve one (or more) personally meaningful goals as purposeful behaviors and related experiences. Symptoms are often complex and ambiguous and can fulfill several purposes in one act of behavior. Symptoms can cope with the unclear and obscure, with contradictory and conflicting motives, symptoms may serve as pseudo-solutions and pacifications without actually grasping or even solving a problem. With regard to the functionality of the symptoms and risk behaviors, there is often a lack of awareness among the patients. Their abilities to detect, reflect on, and verbalize the goals are often very limited at the start of therapy.

The functional context is revealed to the therapist by considering the interactions of the patient with his environment. This approach requires a holistic view [213]. Various types of therapy such as acceptance-and-commitment therapy [214], dialectic-behavioral therapy [215], functional-analytical therapy [216] or mindfulness therapy [217] are subsumed with the term "functional contextualism" [218]. They are summarized and assigned to a so-called third wave of behavior therapy—according to the learning-theory therapy procedures (wave one) and the cognitive turn (wave two)—[213]. A new platform for integrative considerations emerges that allows encounters with developmental psychopathology, which has a completely different tradition, and psychodynamics [219], which genuinely pursues this functional approach with its concept of defense mechanisms and psychological structures (see Chap. 6).

The systemic approach [220] also shows the functionality of symptoms in the interpersonal area in a special way. This chance of a conceptual encounter of different therapeutic approaches and schools of thought on the level of "functional contextualism" should not be missed. Conceptual communication would always keep the differences between the individual approaches in mind. Such a discussion process could consider the necessary flexibility of adolescent psychotherapy more than the rigidity of certain therapy schools and their efforts to differentiate themselves from others even more. From an optimistic point of view, a common basis could be read from different schools and perspectives, which could contribute to the development of a cross-school developmental theory and thus enable an age-appropriate form of treatment, as already expressed in the approaches of "Psychological Therapy" by Grawe [221]. In this way, individually tailored forms of therapy could be developed for adolescents that enable age-appropriate treatment under the umbrella of a uniform developmental theory.

Functional contextualism assumes that the cognitive, emotional and behavioral expressions of the individual can be related to an internal and external context: they gain meaning through biographical and current internal and external events [218]. The patient's behavior must be hermeneutically ascertained. In situational behavioral hermeneutics, the behavior will be read like a text that makes sense in relation to the situation. Seen in this way, there are no objective truths against which the patient's thinking and behavior are measured, but there are contextual-historical insights that suggest each individual his personal truth in the assessment of the world and other people. Thoughts and behaviors always appear to be appropriate and "clever" in relation to the context and not incorrect and false!

Symptoms and risk behaviors must be considered and analyzed together with their context variables and must not be broken down into behavioral blocks in order to be understood as series of causal events one following the other without current environmental relevance. The context must be considered. This is what O'Brien and Carhart [213] call an "in situ" approach.

Hayes (relational frame theory) contrasts behavior controlled by verbal rules with contingency-related behavior, which is shaped by experience (learning through trial and error) in the sense of a differential approach to the environment. All processes of adapting to environmental conditions can be structured in this way. Hayes gives the example of learning to catch a ball or to overcome an obstacle. All types of human behavior based on verbal formulations of events and the relationships between them are referred to as rule-controlled behavior [214]. Narratives of events and contexts can take on the role of rules or reference values. This behavior is controlled more by specifying contingencies than by direct contact with them. Rules may be drawn up by others in order to pass on experiences and to spare the individual negative consequences or dangers and threats. Rules create order. However, rules may also be misused to take control over other people and exercise power over them. In the context of the relationship with caregivers, the children internalize such rules and elevate them to their own goals and mottos. The individual then follows the inner motto rather than the external influences on experience.

Hayes describes three types of rule-controlled behavior through internal verbalization: the first term, "pliance", is derived from the word compliance and defines compliance with a verbal rule that has been internalized through socially mediated consequences. Many educational measures in the child work in this way. The child obeys the rule of the parents, but not because it recognizes the meaning of the rule, but because it wants to satisfy the respective parent, expects praise and anticipates the correctness of the rule for social reasons in the context of attachment (or relies on its meaningfulness). Following rules to satisfy important caregivers leads to the implantation of goals. Prohibitions and commands are conveyed to the child and internalized by the child.

In contrast, "tracking" is a rule-controlled behavior in which the child sees the correspondence between the rule and its consequences in reality. In this context, natural contingencies are important in learning history. It is the way experiences and their narratives shape our memory of rules and goals. In the example of Hayes et al. [214], the child obeys the parental request "Put on a jacket—it's cold outside" not only to satisfy the parents (that would be pliance), but because the child recognizes that it is better to be appropriately dressed in cold temperatures. Many human behaviors can simultaneously serve both one's own horizon of experience and the establishment of relationships with important caregivers. A distinction between the two rules is therefore more functional than formal [214].

"Augmenting" is the third form of rules. Augmenting changes the extent to which an event acts as a consequence. These phenomena can often be observed in advertising. If an adolescent makes the personal experience connecting a certain drink with accentuated male behavior, the personal experience of feeling good and strong when taking such a drink is further enhanced. For example, the advertising of stimulating drinks, which are linked to daring sporting events, has an augmenting effect on the personal motive of taking such drinks. The inner connection between the desire to be sporty and strong and therefore also to turn to the drink does not have to be fully aware.

In clinical contexts, compulsive and rigid types of interactions with the environment may reflect excessive forms of pliance or tracking. Rule-controlled behavior can not only make our relationship with the outside world easier and save us negative consequences, it can also make the contact with the environment dysfunctional. Personal behavior can primarily serve to satisfy others, to receive praise and recognition and to avoid conflicts. As long as personal intent is primarily focused on the relationship aspect, the adolescent can concentrate less on which behaviors could actually be appropriate in the situation. The development of resistance in therapy, which receives special attention in the context of psychodynamic interpretations, can also be represented in this way in a more behavioral concept.

It is important to uncover in adolescents those areas in which behavior loops are maintained even against better knowledge. Findings gained through personal experience such as "I am worthless" or "You must not offend anyone if you are happy or successful" hinder functional adjustments to the respective situation. In psychodynamic therapies, the phase of finding internal contradictions and dysfunctional control loops is called "clarification" [212]. A functional analysis of psychopathological phenomena shows that we are moving in fundamental problem areas of psychotherapy that are also significant beyond the school dispute.

In order to change rule-regulated behaviors, the iconic representations of situations and physical experiences of adolescents often have to be freed from the "corset of language" in therapy. You have to differentiate the naive and pure experience from the inner rules and verbal mottos. The real experience has to be removed from the verbalizations that shape it. The linguistic orders, categories and rules should be pushed back in their power over perception and feeling. Replacing a verbal motto with another verbal motto is often not helpful enough; language may not open up access to experience through language. It is important to create an inner distance between verbal rules and immediate experiences. Words are powerful when they reverberate in us, when parental formulations in us become rules of behavior and inner goals. For too long, upbringing has disciplined young people through words, implemented inner sentences of conscience, and bound experience and behavior to principles and mottos. Honor, responsibility, obedience, faith and other virtues, success, victory and profit have been engraved as inner goals in the developing personalities. Masculinity and femininity, the "you should", the "you must not", the "you have to" stand in the way of young, uncivilized needs. Inner mottos can create feelings of guilt and fear. How can therapy free young people from their straitjackets of education and discipline? How can therapy free young people from the shame of self-degradation?

Verbal inner goals often make young people act against their forebodings and "gut feelings" and against their "better knowledge". The coercion that was external in the upbringing often becomes a motto and self-chosen life goal in later life.

All understanding of environmental contexts, the description and differentiation of feelings, motives and drives ultimately happen through language. Meanings cling to language, narratives shape the memories of any experience. Therapy must free immediate experience and action temporarily from language, it has to open up a space for spontaneity, new formulations and freer mottos can replace the old ones in the aftermath.

We cannot exist as human beings without language. Everything we think is language—except for the things that we develop creatively in action. What we express in pictures, paintings, dances, scenes, figures or sculptures is initially speech-free, so—to free themselves from verbal goals—young people have to go back to action, to design works and create things. Language cannot free from language chains, only action can. Creative self-designs and spontaneous behaviors pave the way for a new linguistic formulation of one's own experience. The creative process of action creates a new awareness of the adolescent's own motives. Thus, inner goals may be changed by new experiences in the light of new relationships.

Chapter 8
Cybernetics and Behavioral Loops

The "cognitive revolution" in behavior therapy (second wave) was the result of scientific developments in the last third of the twentieth century. The focus shifted from observable behavior to mental processes, but the scientific paradigm as a methodology of "chains of causal conclusions" remained unchanged from the beginnings of empirical psychology [222]. Now attempts have been made to map intrapsychic processes in non-linear models and more complex explanatory patterns.

One theory of that time, however, remained relatively unnoticed by the emerging enthusiasm for "cognition", which had already been derived from considerations on cybernetic control loops since the 1950s [223–225]. It is the theory that human behavior is purposeful and can therefore be represented in control loops that were known from mechanical, electrical and electronic engineering. The most notable representative of this theory was W. T. Powers [180]. He called his theory "Perceptual Control Theory". One starting point of Powers is the experience with electrical engineering: "Engineers use negative feedback control systems to hold some physical quantity in a predetermined state, in an environment containing sources of disturbance that tend to change the quantity when it is uncontrolled …" ([226]: 352). In control-system terms, a purpose is not a consequence of behavior, but a model inside the organism for what it wants the perceptual consequences of its outputs to be [226]. "The biggest surprise, of course, is that control systems control their own perceptions, not their output activities. When an organism reacts to some change in external circumstances, the appearance is that of a direct cause-effect relationship. If organisms are control systems, the reality is that between the external phenomenon and the alteration of behavior is a variable affected by both, a controlled quantity or controlled variable being sensed by the organic control system and being held at some reference level by behavior" ([204]: 93). "As an example, consider this observation. I open a window, and a person sitting by the window gets up and puts on a sweater. The appearance is that the sight and sound of the window being opened triggered off a complex series of responses, in a direct cause-effect way. In control-system terms, the relationship is not direct. Opening a window disturbed a

F. Resch, P. Parzer, *Adolescent Risk Behavior and Self-Regulation*,
https://doi.org/10.1007/978-3-030-69955-0_8

controlled quantity, the temperature of the person's skin, and would have disturbed it a lot more if the person had not done something having the opposite effect—put on a sweater. The behavior was protecting a controlled perception against significant disturbance" ([204]: 93).

While scientific psychology is based on the cause-effect model, where a stimulus triggers behavioral responses, the feedback model considers the influence of behavior on future behavior in addition to the stimulus. If behavior is only seen as the consequence of causes, then the purposefulness of behavior is omitted! Evoked behavior is mainly reactive. It may be called "elicited behavior". However, humans mostly do not simply react to disturbances of the environment, they act to withstand such disturbances for the sake of a specific purpose—to reach a goal in spite of this "noise". The variety of behaviors is not due to the variety of environmental influences, but due to the specific obstacles, the environment is setting, on the individual's way to reach a goal. "Emitted behavior" is purposeful behavior.

In the cause-effect model, stimuli act on organisms to produce responses [180]. Powers believes that this venerable model is in error. Responses are dependent on present and past stimuli—this is not to deny. However, it seems equally true, that the effect of stimuli depends on responses according to the actual organization of the environment AND the organism in which the nervous system resides [180]. While behavioral psychology employs an open-loop concept of cause and effect in behavior, the effect (behavior) depends on the cause (stimuli) but not vice versa [180]. The closed-loop concept of Powers treats behavior as one of the causes of that same behavior, so that cause and effect may be traced all the way in a closed loop. The idea of input control in humans means control of perception.

Self-regulation is self-control. The reference level in a given control situation is a property of the organism, not of the environment [204]. An accurate way to describe an organism acting as a good control system is to say that it carries out intentions [204]. An organism as a living system does not directly control the realities of surrounding or environment, it uses information about them. All control—artificial or natural—is organized around a representation of the external state of affairs [204].

Not more not less. However, behavioral critique has argued that the model of behavior as a closed loop between input and output is simply too mechanistic, "... in that the components of the feedback loop are analyzed as unidirectional, linear causal chain ... there is no dialectic interpenetration, or reciprocal interaction, because ... the components are inseparable from the whole or structure that comprises them." ([227]: 1119). Up to recent years, there has been a hindrance against the adoption of this model for the explanation of pathological behavior. Why? Is it too simplistic on one hand and too complex in the mathematical formulation on the other?

However, the model directs our explanations of risk behaviors from causation of behavior through brain functions or from causation of behavior by environmental stimuli to the focus on goal-directed behavior. The model still directs our focus away from the nowadays mainstream explanations of behavior. Behavior tries to serve intentions, motives and goals. Behavior does not simply follow brain circuit's processes like a slave and behavior does not simply answer to stimuli. Behavior may be conditioned operantly—but only when the reinforcement fits the individual's goals and needs.

The thoughts were later taken up by C. S. Carver and M. F. Scheier and used to explain the self-regulation of behavior in humans [228]. Further attempts at implementation in practice were made by R. S. Marken [229], W. Mansell [230] and T. A. Carey [231].

This theory of regulation of human behavior fits perfectly into the developmental psychopathology paradigm of adolescent risk behavior and is a consequent implementation of the cybernetic interpretations for the emergence of such behavior in the development process. The theory will be briefly explained below:

According to control loop theory, targeted human behavior can be represented like a cybernetic circle. As has been already mentioned, we recognize control loops for example in electronic components, or in automatic room temperature regulation using thermostats. In biology, control loops are used to explain the reaction principle in the fine-tuning of muscular activities, or to understand neuroendocrine mechanisms such as stress regulation by corticoids in the Hypothalamus-Pituitary-Adrenal System (HPA-axis) [232].

The hypothalamic-pituitary-adrenal cortex (HPA)-system is the central complex hormonal system for the adaptation of the organism to physical or psychological stressors. The endocrine stress response is constructed in the form of a negative feedback loop: The peripheral agent is cortisol. The steroid hormone cortisol is released into the blood from the adrenal cortex. Cortisol exerts its effect on the target organs via specific receptors and increases the energy availability in the acute stress response. Glucose is newly synthesized and mobilized from glycogen, lipolysis is increased and the availability of amino acids is increased. In addition to an increase in heart strength, blood pressure is also increased. Suppression is exerted on the immune system. Since cortisol cannot be stored in large amounts in the adrenal cortex, the synthesis of the hormone is increased if necessary. The stimulating adreno-corticotrope-hormone (ACTH) promotes synthesis and release.

ACTH is produced in the pituitary gland and secreted into the bloodstream, which brings it to the adrenal gland. The activities of ACTH are stimulated by the corticotropin-releasing hormone (CRH), which is released by the hypothalamus and controls the ACTH synthesis and release of the pituitary gland. CRH itself is stimulated by stressors that affect the brain. In particular, situations of uncontrollability, insecurity and social threats act as corresponding stressors.

ACTH also has peripheral effects on attention, concentration and has a generally activating effect. Cortisol exerts a feedback effect on the pituitary gland and therefore slows down its stimulation when released. There is also an effect on the hypothalamus, mitigating the stress-induced reference value. The actual reference value is set in the hypothalamus. The feedback loop brings the HPA-axis back into balance after a temporary increase in the reference value and keeps it in a physiological range. The necessary level of the hormone cortisol is measured in the pituitary gland and regulated by ACTH. The goal is given by the hypothalamus.

The behavioral control loop consists of the same elements as technical or biological control loops. It starts with a target—which is also quantitatively referred to as a reference level. This goal is to be achieved and maintained. A behavioral response is set in motion by a comparator, which detects the current deviations from the target level or reference level, which sets in motion the behavioral reaction to exert an effect on the environment—in order to bring about a suitable change. This change is then fed back into the comparator via a perception process to recognize and monitor the current approach or distance to the target (reference level) (see Fig. 8.1). As long as the target value—the reference level—is not reached, the behavior is maintained, i.e. the effort to change the environment in favor of the target remains active. Strictly speaking, the individual acts in the control loop in order to change his perception of the environment in such a way that the goal is achieved or approximated as possible. The key to achieving the goal is therefore not just the behavioral effect on the environment, but the knowledge of an environmental change—however, this is caused by behavior or other factors—which then interrupts the behavior.

Purposeful behaviors—and many, if not all, human activities show this pattern—can be better explained by control loops (closed loops) than by a causal chain (open loop), the end of which is the behavioral response, which then exerts an effect on the environment as an answer to the stimulus [222]. Closed loops are able to explain behaviors that follow a specific purpose within a given environment. Furthermore, only the control loop theory makes it possible to explain why behaviors are often maintained against better knowledge and against the challenges of the environment, if this is the only way to pursue an internal goal or to meet a personal need. It makes the maintenance of perspectives, the immunization of attitudes and evaluations, an "unsuitable" fit in spite of existing counter-information explainable. Unreasonable,

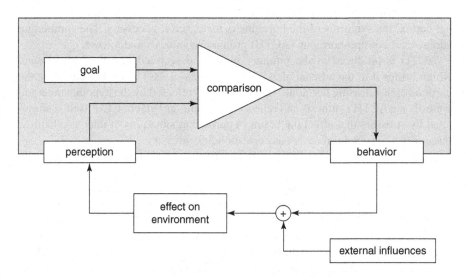

Fig. 8.1 Behavior and perception constitute the feedback loop of human adaptation

emotionally guided and apparently "illogical" behavior can be explained in a logical way, because the behavior is not related to the environment, but to internal goals. Even a "tendentious apperception" [233], i.e. the emotionally changed perception of the environment "distorted" by inner goals for personal goal achievement—as it is formulated in individual psychology [234]—makes sense in this way and gains a meaning of adaptation.

However, human behavior cannot be fully understood in a single control loop. That would be too simple. Many—often contradicting—goals, motives, wishes, tendencies and appetites guide spontaneous human behavior. Powers [180] and Carver and Scheier [228] therefore construct complex behaviors from hierarchically nested control loops, each of which pursues a specific—superordinate or subordinate—behavioral goal (see Fig. 8.2). Following this view, a resulting behavioral response can ultimately serve many hierarchical goals. The details of the model would far exceed the scope of this book and can be read in the book by Carver and Scheier [228]. The control loop theory provides a good explanatory framework for functional symptom analyses.

On the other hand, if the goal of the behaviorist methodology is to find environmental variables (stimuli) that causally influence behavior, then the goal of a cybernetic view of behavior is to find those target values and motives that are regulated by behavior as reference values [222]. In the view of causal chains, the behavior is caused by internal and/or external influences and per se without a goal, simply answering to changes of the environment. In the control loop model, the behavior serves to influence one's own perceptions of the environmental conditions in such a

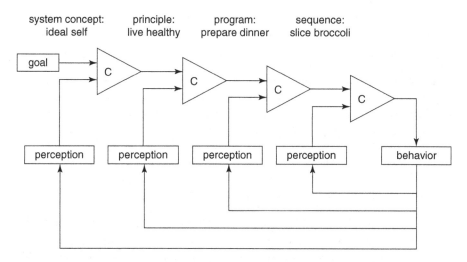

Fig. 8.2 Example of a hierarchy of control loops (adapted from [180, 228]). A person with an idealized sense of self tries to be in line with the principle of health behavior, presently being realized by the act of preparing dinner, which involves a series of action sequences including the cutting up of broccoli for steaming. Each systems output becomes the reference value for the next system and is compared (C) with the actual perception of this hierarchy level

way that they approximate the internal reference level—the goal. That is a fundamental difference!

However, in the functional view according to the control loop model, we cannot directly deduce any biological or experience-related causes from a problem behavior, but rather have to ask which internal goals this behavior is going to obey, what purposes it serves for the person, what internal motives are regulated by it. The restriction to diagnostic categories is not helpful for the search for an intervention based on the functional analysis of behavior—if a control loop of behavior and motives is suspected at the center! The same psychopathological phenomena can be subject to very different goals for the person (e.g. self-esteem stabilization, search for identity, desire for recognition and self-affirmation, needs for motive replacement or motivational conflicts). However, such internal goals can contribute to the maintenance of symptoms and lead to therapy-failure if they are not observed and payed attention to. Various different symptoms can serve the same goals. This explains why many adolescents experience symptom shifts between different risk behaviors and often present a changing variety of symptoms.

Symptoms that cannot be easily changed by interventions indicate controlled behaviors (e.g. in the case of depression or anorexia). This non-change is actively maintained and costs a lot of strength and energy. Varying impulses for change should be tried out in the therapeutic context and can only challenge the system of symptoms and internal goals again and again from different directions. If the problem behavior persistently does not change, this indicates that this problem behavior is regulated by an internal guideline and its reference level is maintained as resistance against all interventions for an important purpose. Apparently, the problem behavior still serves the goal best and is not being released. In order to bring about a change in behavior, an alternative solution must be found for this benchmark, this inner goal (e.g. keeping self-esteem stable). Only then the problem behavior can stop. The search for alternatives must go hand in hand with the symptom treatment following the functional considerations.

Basically, there is no point in deriving individual motifs as specific to certain psychopathological syndromes. For example, ascriptions of "wanting to remain a child" or "not wanting to become an adult woman" have not been empirically confirmed in anorexia nervosa patients as typical core motifs. Even the motivational spectrum in self-harm and self-injury is highly diverse and not uniform. You can't deduce the motive from the symptom! Symptoms and risk behaviors serve various goals.

Control loop models can be extended from the individual level to the level of families and transactional systems. Individual control loop hierarchies can be integrated as individual elements in groups of such systems. The control loop model is therefore not only applicable to the individual patient, but can also be applied to social systems, as is done in the theory-building of systemic therapy [220]. However, systemic paradigms do not strictly follow the cybernetic rules of perception control theory. For the individual, social systems form the complex environment that affects them and in which they strive to achieve their goals and motives.

Caregivers and their goals thus represent the social environments of the individual. The more ambiguous and contradictory the rules in these environments, the more impenetrable the environment, the more difficult it is for the individual to find his way around when he tries to coordinate his needs with the environmental conditions. Early experiences of interaction create a canon of experiences in the individual that allows more or less predictions and suggests solutions for contradictions and problems. The schema therapy [235] makes explicit reference to these early experiences and tries to change the resulting limitations of coping in the "here and now".

The control loop model allows the internal goals to be systematically recorded in their current form, in particular to be inferred from the situational behavior and experience. It is therefore not solely dependent on the conscious verbal self-reports, which only rarely reveal the actual "hidden goals" and which can be altered or "beautified" by social desirability or lack of transparency, if they are accessible to conscious self-reflection at all. Current experiences and behavior can be compared with biographical behavioral accents and classified in a context of the meaning of the life span. Not only what someone says and verbally claims, but what someone does and how he behaves reflects his thinking. What someone expresses in his instantaneous actions forms the material for hermeneutic efforts in the sense of "behavioral hermeneutics". Risk behaviors may be explained by their meaningful purposes.

8.1 Experiment to Illustrate a Control Loop

To illustrate the interdependency between goals, environmental conditions, and behavior, the following experiment is introduced. In this experiment, behavior is looked at from the point of view of *form* and *function*. An adolescent trying to upgrade self-worth and identity feelings by risky behavior can be interpreted as follows: The risk behavior is the *form* of the behavior; the impact on the self is the *function* of the behavior.

The following simple experiment demonstrates the difference between *form* and *function* of behavior. In the control task, the subject is instructed to keep a red dot on the computer screen as close as possible to the center of the screen marked by a white cross. The position of the dot can be changed by moving the computer mouse, but a computer-generated random process simulates an environmental disturbance invisible to the subject, that is added to the mouse position. To keep the dot close to the cross, the subject has to compensate the disturbance by moving the mouse. The control task is thus a model of a two-dimensional control loop. If the random process generated by the computer is a slowly moving random walk, then it is not too difficult for the subject to keep the dot close to the cross. Figure 8.3 shows one exemplary result of this task. To simplify the presentation only the vertical positions are plotted. The horizontal positions are similar.

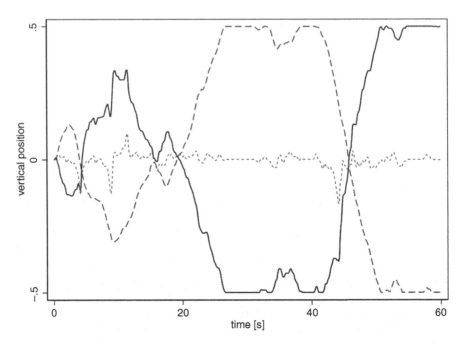

Fig. 8.3 Vertical positions of the mouse (solid line), disturbance (dashed line), and dot (dotted line) against time for an exemplary run of the control task. The cross is at position 0

A striking aspect of the Fig. 8.3 is that the mouse position (solid line) mirrors the computer-generated random walk (dashed line). This is a logical consequence of the control loop. To keep the dot near the cross, the subject has to compensate the movement of the disturbance by moving the mouse in the opposite direction. The dotted line, depicting the vertical position of the dot, is most of the time close to zero, the vertical position of the cross, showing that the subject is quite successful in controlling the position of the dot. Since the position of the dot is the sum of the positions of the disturbance and the mouse, the mouse position is closely mirroring the disturbance.

This simple task exemplifies an important characteristic of control loops. If control is successful then the *form* of behavior is completely determined by the environment. The form of the behavior tells us nothing about the subject, but everything about the environment. What tells us something about the subject is the *function* of the behavior. We see in Fig. 8.3, that the function of the behavior is to keep the dot close to the cross. This tells us, that the subject followed the instructions of the task.

In a more demanding version of the control task, the effect of the mouse is inverted at some point during the experiment. That means, that the dot moves downwards if the mouse is moved upward, to the right if the mouse is moved to the left

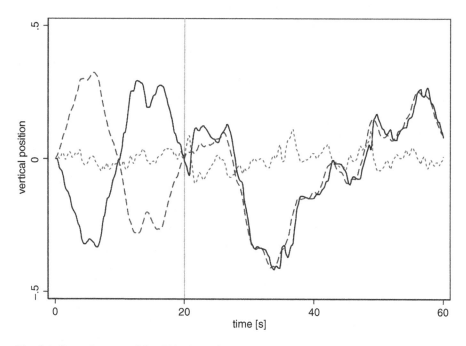

Fig. 8.4 Exemplary run of the difficult version of the control task. At the time indicated by the gray vertical line the effect of the mouse is inverted

and vice versa. The position of the dot is now the position of the disturbance minus the position of the mouse. An exemplary result of the difficult version of the control task is shown in Fig. 8.4.

After some short irritation, the subject learns very fast the new rules and keeps the dot again quite near the cross, albeit not as good as in the easy version of the task. Now the position of the mouse follows the position of the disturbance since the position of the dot is the position of the disturbance minus the position of the mouse.

By changing the rules of the environment, we learn something about the subject. We learn, that this subject can adapt to changes in the environment. But again, we do not learn this by looking at the *form* of the behavior. The form of the behavior is again determined by the environment. We learn this by observing, that the subject can regain control of the position of the dot even after changes in the rules of the environment.

Such a sudden change of the rules of the environment does not happen in the physical world, but in social environments such changes are common. If an adolescent has to change school, then a behavior, that made the adolescent popular in one school, can have the opposite effect in another school.

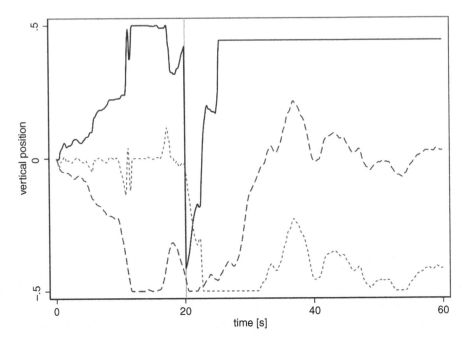

Fig. 8.5 Result of the difficult version of the control task for a subject that could not adapt to the inversion of the mouse effect. The sudden movement of the mouse at the time of switching the mouse effect is an artifact of the program. The prevent a jump of the dot when inverting the mouse effect, the coordinates of the mouse position are changed in a such way that the dot stays the at the same position

Figure 8.5 shown an example of a subject, that could not adapt to the change of the rules in the difficult version of the control task.

After the inversion of the mouse effect, the subject still tries to move the dot towards the cross by the same behavior as before the switch, causing the dot to move away from the cross. After a few seconds, the subject believes, that it has lost control over the dot and stops moving the mouse at all. The subject withdraws from the situation.

If the reader wants to try the experiment by himself, the code can be downloaded from https://github.com/pparzer/control.

Chapter 9
Functional Symptom Analysis

In the functional symptom analysis, an attempt is made to combine the control loop model with the concepts of "psychic structures" [142, 236] and Grawe's principle of consistency to explain mental disorders [221].

If we take the control loop as a basis, we can highlight four aspects that impair the functionality of the experience and action of our patients:

- The ability to act, the emitting of behavior, may be limited in the light of the goal, i.e. the behavioral output may not take place in an appropriate manner. If the achievement of goals demands a certain achievement from the adolescent, which cannot be fulfilled by the behavioral performance, (e.g. in the case of physical impairment and athletic goals, lack of talent in artistic goals or requests for communication with others and social phobia) the control loop for maintaining the goal of action, the strive for sport or artistic success, the strive for contact and affirmation remains active. Such activities can be repeated until, for example, overarching goals—such as self-esteem which longs to be increased by the success of the subordinate control loop—collapse or seek compensation in other behaviors (e.g. internet use or drug abuse) or turn to another form of self-protection in symptoms of self-harm.
- Deficits in perception can also make control loops dysfunctional. If the input is inadequate, a possible change in the environment towards the behavioral goal cannot be processed by the internal comparator. Deficits in "feeling" and in the perception of emotions or distortions of perception due to inappropriate affects can keep the control loop unduly active. It is therefore not only important to bring about appropriate behavioral consequences in the environment in order to achieve the goal, but also to sharpen the perception in order to be able to recognize corresponding environmental changes. If you don't compute the changes in the environment caused by your behavior, then your comparator will still be highly active and signals further necessary efforts.

F. Resch, P. Parzer, *Adolescent Risk Behavior and Self-Regulation*,
https://doi.org/10.1007/978-3-030-69955-0_9

- Control loops can also get out of hand if they are driven by an "impossible to reach" target value (reference level). There may be unrealistic expectations of the person (like in our first example) or internal conflicts in the target hierarchies (wanting something which the moral system does not allow) that make it impossible to achieve the reference value from the outset. This can result in senselessly perpetuated activities.
- Control loops can also remain overactive due to a defect in the comparator. If discrepancies between the target value and current behavior are exaggerated in the wrong way, the control loop remains active, even if the target level has already been reached. An over-perfectionism, which still requires more accuracy, more precision and confirmation when approximating the target value, can result in exaggerated behavior.

Based on the thesis that symptoms and risk behaviors always express a lack of consistency between internal conditions and external requirements [221], that they address the problem of an imbalance between challenges and resources, that symptoms and risk behaviors show an incompatibility of goals, motives, experiences and behavior under particular environmental conditions, we propagate four diagnostic steps of a functional symptom analysis [57]. These diagnostic steps are intended to illuminate the adaptive function of the symptoms and risk behaviors. The functional analysis starts with some basic questions:

- Can current symptoms and behaviors not only cause suffering and disrupt adaptation, but also help to solve a person's problem at another level?
- Can symptoms in a family context interrupt unbearable tensions and conflicts of the person or the whole family?
- What could be achieved through symptoms and risk behaviors in a particular person?

In contrast, classical psychopathology always draws attention to the aspects of what the patient cannot achieve with his symptoms or that certain goals are rendered impossible by the symptoms.

- How much is a current symptom accentuated by disaster tendencies and escalation loops in the interaction with important others?
- Is there an aggravation loop (e.g. fear of fear) in the self-assessment of individual symptoms and the resulting psychological consequences?
- Can symptoms contribute disease gains?
- Which goals do the current experiences and behaviors serve, postponing the question of where the symptoms come from in the sense of a causal derivation?

The *first step* is to examine the relationship between symptoms and *environmental conditions*. The symptoms cannot be assessed regardless of the situational context (Chap. 7). Are symptoms complicating a fundamentally respectful and relatively positive social environment? Or do the symptoms relate to a demanding or overwhelming environment, as can be noted in traumatic situations? Patient's behavior can be a normal response to an unmanageable environment! Many examples from adolescent psychotherapy follow this pattern: Under traumatizing conditions, symptoms are sensible answers and "cries for help" to an overwhelming, perfidious or pathological environment in the family, school or social neighborhood. A conflictual or traumatizing environment can systematically prevent the achievement of internal goals. If the symptoms appear as an expression of an unsuccessful attempt to adapt in unclear or recognizable dangerous environmental conditions, or as a pathological compromise for survival in a hostile environment, the therapeutic approach must first be dedicated to securing patients in the present. Psychotherapy should not encourage the perpetuation of traumatizing conditions and make "the unbearable endurable". In such a case, the therapeutic interventions should primarily focus on improving the environmental conditions, which enables the patient to be protected, assisted and vitally secured. The adolescents need support against emotional or physical abuse and sexual assault, they must be brought to safety in an emergency. The therapeutic location must primarily be a refuge. Disasters that affect patients and their families as a whole (such as war events, environmental disasters or accidents) need help and support for the families. The strengthening of the caregivers can help to start coping processes in the families and thus indirectly influence the adolescents therapeutically.

A *second* diagnostic *step* checks the *target values* in detail. What are the goals, the reference levels of current behavior? What sense do the current symptoms have in the overall context when you consider the central motives for action? This diagnostic step is particularly demanding because the goals are not immediately verbally told and must be developed hermeneutically from behavior in context—against the background of biographical knowledge. Like in the theatre, there are always individual themes, as mottos on stage, that open the space for new scenes when they are recognized. The work is directed from the surface of the common and (self-) understandable to even deeper goals, which the patient can only discover in the diagnostic-therapeutic work. Recognizing the hidden goals of action is fundamentally important. Because if the immediate target values and reference levels are unattainable or even dysfunctional (e.g. "you always have to be successful" or "you always have to act in such a way that you satisfy your counterpart"), you have to advance to the next higher level in the control loop hierarchy to eliminate possible contradictions: the model of hierarchical control loops is designed in such a way that each target value is set by the output of a higher control loop in the hierarchy. Only a consistent hierarchy of goals can be achieved within the framework of regulated behavior.

Contradicting or unrealistically unattainable goals make targeted effective adaptation to the environment impossible. What is the relationship between target value and emotional reaction (alarm)? Conflicting goals, conflicting motives and inconsistent hierarchies of goals can exhaust the individual internally and induce behaviors that radiate inappropriately into the environment without calming down or making changes. Are there persistent conflicts in dealing with important life issues? Does the individual finally reach his biological limits in excessive actions? Also, insights that set the motto "I am worthless—no success can hide this" or "You must not offend anyone by doing well and must always weigh up your own wishes" or

"You have to assert yourself—but asserting yourself is always dangerous and will lead to rejection by others" hinder functional adjustments to the respective situation. Such a motto stands in the way of developing one's own needs and hinders constructive actions to deal with current problems. For some people, the goals come out clearly in acted out behaviors. In others, the goals remain locked in a mental space and can only be inferred indirectly from sparse actions in the everyday context. The question remains: What does the person who presents himself with these symptoms really want to achieve, what does he show in the current context, what is he aiming at? What future is the person aiming for? Or has the individual closed for itself with the future and only acts in the immediate present?

We should not forget: The discussion about goals of behavior, about motives and target values—that should be achieved—must not deceive us. Man is not a rational being who pursues clear conscious goals. Rather, people are strongly irrational, driven by emotions and captivated by security needs, self-worth problems or sexual appetite. In addition, there are the mottos and guiding ideas from the upbringing. Parents have left their mark on young people through the implantation of goals. That means: the "goals" we postulate and are looking for are not crystalline, reasonable thoughts. They are the results of deep currents and irrational—often unconscious—guidelines. They become more recognizable in behavior than in personal comments or arguments.

In the *third step*, the effort to adapt to the current problem has to be checked: Is the emitted behavior successful? Does it serve the goals expressed by patients and their parents, does it solve the indicated problem? Or does it run counter to the framework conditions, does it perpetuate itself because it serves other (former) goals and is concerned with tasks that have been successfully accomplished before? Behavior can become rigid if there is a lack of feedback. Validation may be required to remove "learning fatigue". Recourse to previously successful strategies does not currently have to be successful. It is important to work out changes in one's own experience and behavior within the framework of relationships. In the old learning theories, such learning processes were initiated by "shaping". Psychoanalysis [219] and schema therapy [235] also conceptualized this problem and worked out therapeutic options. In complex form, we are trying today to initiate social-emotional learning processes on an individual and family level that help the personal emancipation of adolescents with regard to their problem environment. Does the adolescent present with internalized behavioral goals and overriding mottos from past relationship contexts that prevent mastering of current life tasks? In clinical contexts, compulsive and rigid types of interactions with the environment can be identified if, for example, personal behavior is primarily geared towards satisfying others, receiving praise and recognition and avoiding interactional conflicts. As long as personal intent is primarily focused on the relationship aspect, the adolescents can concentrate less freely on which actions might actually be appropriate in the situation. It is important to discover overarching mottos, such as basic knowledge of "I want this—but I will not be able to gain it anyway", can weaken efforts to act from the outset. Rigid adjustment schemes as a result of emotional experiences or sensitizations that have arisen in previous life situations (similar to the allergy processes at the immunological level) can make current experiences and behavior excessive and/ or dysfunctional. Such motivational and behavioral restrictions—once recognized and worked out—then apply to the therapy focus.

The *fourth* diagnostic *step* deals with the issues of the structural integrity of the regulatory system of the self: are there fundamental defects in self-regulation? Are there structural deficits in the self-system? Or even more basic "tool failures" in cognitive processing and reality testing? Are there defects in the perception system? Can the individual recognize the environment appropriately in his own social perception? Or is this perception distorted by wishes or discrepant motives? Then the target hierarchy has to be checked again. Assimilatory activities of self-deception can allegedly achieve goals, although the conditions in the environment would still require adaptation (wish-fulfillment through perceptual distortion or imaginary solutions). However, social perception can also be fundamentally impaired (in the sense of a disorder of basic functions), as we know from the treatment of children from the autistic spectrum, or can be complicated by perceptual disorders (acoustic hallucinations), which we have to consider in psychotherapy for schizophrenic psychoses. Further structural disturbances of the person in the domains of their relationships, their internal representations, their self-awareness, their self-reflection and their self-control (lack of impulse control) can prevent the adolescent from performing his life at any age and make developmental tasks impossible [47]. The therapeutic answer to this is, for example, structural psychotherapy [236], or the use of other therapeutic measures that are already established for "disorders of psychic structure" and "borderline disorders", and to be able to offer the patients support in their self-regulatory processes.

Interventions should relate to those areas where change seems possible and necessary. If we look at the environment of adolescents, many families sometimes do not seem so unfavorable for them despite the high dysfunctionality of their communication patterns because they allow changes in behavior at all. On the other hand, in facade families that seem completely normal to the outside, there is so little room for maneuver for the adolescents that they do not find a "way out" of the family context. The chance of change is therefore not a question of global dysfunctionality of systems, but of the dysfunctionality that is particularly important for the individual. The concept of a fit between the individuals and their social environment is functionally significant.

Using the control loop paradigm, it is possible to intervene simultaneously in different fields or domains of the bio-psycho-social model without losing sight of the overarching goal. Such multimodal interventions do not correspond to helpless polypragmasia ("intervening in many fields helps a lot"), but all interventions serve a common rational therapeutic goal. They serve to optimize the function of the behavior-related dynamic system.

The control loop paradigm allows the recognition and assignment of experiences and behaviors to one or more internal goals. Even the self-immunization of ideas, selective perception, adherence to a fixed idea, the central setting of a life motto against better knowledge can thus be explained by the paradigm of perceptional control theory. Also, phenomena of mass suggestion, the narrow-mindedness to believe in something that reason recognizes as impossible, the seductiveness through advertising and populism, the psychological stress through group membership and peer pressure correspond to internal goals that are maintained and served by behavior and perception. They might be consolidated even by untruths, "alternative facts" or fiction, if these fit the goal. Inner goals can be set as mottos through education by care persons (see Chap. 7). Last but not least, even delusions serve a goal, representing an uncorrectable explanation for extraordinary experiences and perceptions, even hallucinations serve internal objectives and are contextually integrated. Addictive behaviors revolve around central life issues and wishes. Basic needs define behavioral goals. Sheer reason cannot go against them. To change habits means to change behavior. To change behavior means to change goals.

"People believe what they want to believe ... You can provide them with facts, you can refute them, it doesn't help. On the contrary, if someone wants to believe something, he will find a way! He will squeeze through the tiny gap that the truth leaves him ..." ([237]: 171, translated by the authors).

A few clinical examples are intended to illustrate these facts [57]:

A 13-year-old female patient continues to gain weight as part of the treatment of her anorexia nervosa. The weight curve hardly approaches the target weight when the patient begins to lose weight again. Anorectic behavior returns, resistance to treatment becomes clear. A functional context analysis reveals particular relationships with the parents. The parents, whose partner relationship reveals profound disharmony and conflicting disputes, had reunited around their daughter's life-threatening illness and looked after the therapy attempts, the cooperation with the therapists and the recovery steps in a caring manner. However, when an improvement of their daughter came within reach, the partner conflicts began to escalate again and a desire to separate came out clearly, which burdened the girl very much. Due to the renewed weight loss and an increase in worries on the part of the parents, the idea of separation of the parents was temporarily averted and joint care was guaranteed. Such functional mechanisms can only be recognized and resolved if the adolescent is viewed in a family context and analyzed "in situ". The parent issue and the adolescent's fear can then be addressed therapeutically and the different needs clarified and decoupled. Only when the parents can resolve their conflict independently of the girl's illness at the couple level can the patient's recovery be released from the fatal functionality in the family context.

Another 15-year-old patient with anorexia nervosa also showed late resistance to the therapy after initial therapy progress with weight gain and improvements in mood, when she came closer to the target weight. In the therapy dialogues, she expressed fears of what she would still be when her special role as anorexic girl no longer defined her life. Whether she would still be noticed at all, or whether she would drown completely as a "gray mouse" in an anonymous crowd of her peers. This worry about a lack of peculiarity, a loss of attention by others after taking off the "life-threatening thinness" patient role, dominated her thoughts. She didn't want to drop the role of the anorectic patient until she could otherwise appear as a unique and notable person. If such subjective meanings of symptoms are ignored in therapy, it may be that the problem behavior is fixed in a control loop and maintained against all therapy attempts. Creative therapy methods such as art therapy, music therapy, dance therapy or other possibilities for self-opening can bring the patients to new dimensions of their self, make talents visible and have a self-stabilizing effect.

A young female patient from Kosovo (14 years) suffered from bulimia nervosa. Despite a good therapeutic relationship and active participation in the therapies, her symptoms did not want to stop. A functional analysis of the overall situation showed that the patient's family was threatened with deportation. The family in Germany should only be tolerated while the girl was still in therapy. Thus there were great family needs to maintain the symptoms and the therapy context. In her family solidarity, the adolescent experienced so much pressure that she could not let go of the symptom.

Self-injury symptoms (non-suicidal self-injury, NSSI) comprising cuts in the arms or legs served to relieve internal tension in a 16-year-old patient, relieving emotional pressure and relieving the feeling of "going insane" due to her problems. On the other hand, the patient regularly showed her cuts to the adults in the ward and wanted everyone to be able to see how badly she was actually doing. At the verbal level, she shared her negative thoughts and feelings very sparingly. Therapy procedures aimed at stopping self-harm should also enable alternative strategies to control strong emotions and should not only focus on symptom elimination. Only when the present is secured and no threatening behavior endangers the patient's center of life, can a traumatic past be reappraised in the light of a future orientation. We therefore assume that self-harm represents a form of self-regulation. The body becomes a matrix of self-harming actions that serve to care for other parts of the self. In this way, the self tries to maintain its life competence. The narcissistic anger is channeled, the depersonalization is ended and the self-harm is made tangible as an identity-creating act. In contrast, it can be shown that self-harm on the interpersonal level can send an urgent appeal to the environment and serve to re-enact traumatic situations and intrapsychic dilemmas [95].

Causal thinking (which dysfunction or environmental trigger has elicited this behavior?) seems to be blind to the context and functionality of symptoms. Functional thinking is particularly important when causally oriented forms of therapy (e.g. drugs) remain unsuccessful. In the case of therapy failure in particular, it is therefore important to take the functionality of contexts into account. Several examples were given in which a regulated behavior opposed the success of the therapy. In this way—as our examples show—self-esteem and identity problems can thwart weight gain in anorexic girls. Fears of what life could look like without the special role of anorexia nervosa, who would the patient be if she was completely lost as a gray mouse in an anonymous crowd of her peers? Concern about a lack of specificity and uniqueness, about the loss of attention by others, can dominate the minds of patients in such a way that they cannot give up the role of anorexics.

Being sick or being healthy is embedded in a social framework that is shaped by the mental state of the adolescents. The effects on the social environment can impair individual therapeutic effects.

Functional psychopathology becomes more important where therapeutic interventions are to take place on several levels in the bio-psycho-social model. The combination of drug-therapy and psychotherapeutic procedures requires a link between the different bio-psycho-social viewing levels of humans.

Socio-therapeutic measures and family interventions try to create room for development in which psychological changes in the patient can actually manifest. In contrast, psychotherapeutic procedures are able to both create a safe place and serve to clarify motives and fantasies and to make experience and behavior more flexible, as they can help to compensate for structural, mental and regulatory deficits of the self.

Psychotherapeutic work relies heavily on functional aspects of symptoms in the current environment. In the combination therapy of psychotherapy and pharmacotherapy, the causal and final considerations of the person are not opposed to each other, they are not mutually exclusive, but can complement each other for the benefit of the patient [57].

There are 5 key statements about the treatment of risk behaviors [57]:

- Psychotherapy in adolescents can not only be based on nosological considerations.
- The reduction of self-harming and stressful symptoms requires a structural analysis of the resources of the adolescent.
- An individual functional symptom analysis is based on functional contextualism.
- Cybernetic views of behavior based on the control loop model allow bio-psycho-social functional symptom analysis.
- The cybernetic view of the clinical symptoms allows a better allocation of individual therapeutic interventions in the bio-psycho-social model.

Chapter 10
New Morbidity and Zeitgeist

10.1 New Morbidity and Psychological Symptom Prevalence

The "New Morbidity in Childhood and Adolescence" is a term for different disorders that have become the focus of public attention in recent decades. Since the serious infectious diseases of childhood through vaccinations and antibiotics have lost their horror and since childhood cancer and congenital metabolic disorders, as well as congenital malformations, could be contained through early detection and treatment, new clinical pictures have occupied the treatment area. According to Schlack and Brockmann [238], these are in the narrower sense emotional and behavioral problems, functional disorders such as developmental disorders of language, problems of cognitive and motor skills, obesity and eating disorders as well as other risk behaviors like substance abuse and addictive behavior. In a broader sense, chronic somatic clinical pictures are also attributed to new morbidity, with the allergic diseases being particularly noteworthy here. The new morbidity has led to a shift in the focus of the disease spectra prevailing in childhood and adolescence since the 1960s [238].

After the great progress of medical treatment in childhood and adolescence, a shift manifested itself in the pediatric field: from primarily physical illnesses to disorders of functional and psychological development as well as from acute to the more chronic diseases. If one follows the pediatric authors, the new morbidity disorders are particularly noteworthy for their epidemic clustering. The malfunctions as such had always existed, but they had remained more in the background in previous decades. Since children who suffer from disorders in the context of new morbidity are ultimately not able to bring their individual developmental potential to bloom, the above-mentioned disorders are of particular relevance to social medicine [238] and developmental psychopathology [35].

In the following we want to concentrate more on risk behaviors and the emotional disorders and ask whether there has actually been an increase in mental and psychosocial problems in recent decades. An overview of 41 prevalence studies

F. Resch, P. Parzer, *Adolescent Risk Behavior and Self-Regulation*, https://doi.org/10.1007/978-3-030-69955-0_10

from 27 countries [3] shows a pooled prevalence of mental disorders in children and adolescents of 13.4% (confidence interval 11.3–15.9). Thus, in this meta-analysis, the global prevalence of anxiety disorders is specified with 6.5% (confidence interval 4.7–9.1), of depressive disorders with 2.6% (confidence interval 1.7–3.9), of attention deficit Hyperactivity disorders (ADHD) with 3.4% (confidence interval 2.6–4.5) and of all behavioral disorders with 5.7% (confidence interval 4.0–8.1). A large heterogeneity was found in all pooled estimates [3].

The longitudinal Bella study [239] on 1255 children and adolescents showed significant psychological problems in 10.4% in the initial examination. In the follow-up examination after 1 year 11.2%, in the two-year follow-up 10.6% significant psychological abnormalities could be shown. At the time of the six-year follow-up, it was 10.2%. If one focuses on the entire six-year period, it can be seen that 7.3% of children and adolescents had acute or recurring mental health problems. 2.9% had persistent problems and 15.5% had returned to normal. Overall, 25.7% of the children in the six-year period were affected by a psychological problem! [239].

The question of an increase in mental disorders in recent decades has also been addressed in several studies. An overview by Barkmann and Schulte-Markwort [240] concludes that the prevalence of psychological abnormalities among children and adolescents in Germany is 17.2%. In the context of this overview, an increase or decrease in psychological abnormalities in childhood and adolescence over the decades cannot be derived. However, the reviews by Atladottir et al. [241] and Collishaw [45], based on meta-analyzes of recent literature, conclude that there is a secular trend of increasing emotional problems and anti-social behavior among children and adolescents in highly developed industrial countries. Periods of increases and decreases in individual symptom prevalence are reported. The evidence for countries with middle and low incomes is only limited. Attention Deficit Hyperactivity Disorder (ADHD) showed no evidence of a systematic rise in frequency, but there was an increasing tendency for depressive disorders to begin in adolescence [45]. Emotional problems in adolescence seem to have increased significantly in several European countries over the past 30 years. This increase appears to be greater for girls than for male adolescents. There is a significant intercultural variation in the prevalence of mental health problems in that children of developing countries are significantly more exposed to mental disorders. Increasing numbers were also documented for sleep problems in children, fatigue syndrome and somatic complaints. Significant increases are also evident in self-injuries and suicide attempts in several highly developed countries [242]. In the summary of existing evidence, one must assume an increase in emotional and behavioral problems in childhood and adolescence over the past decades!

10.2 Prevalence Increase in Risk Behaviors?

There are three arguments for an only ostensible increase in the prevalence of mental disorders, which will be discussed below:

A first argument is the increasing willingness in society to recognize, diagnose and treat mental disorders in recent decades. This increased "awareness" for psychological problems in childhood and adolescence allows to identify, name and treat particular disorders in adolescents, who previously had to suffer from undefinable disturbances of their development. In this way, previously undiscovered mental disorders in children and adolescents now have become evident in various countries, from which an apparent increase in overall prevalence can be derived [241]. However, this explanation cannot fundamentally satisfy all questions about prevalence increases. Collishaw [45] gives several reasons that recognizing and reporting symptoms alone cannot be held responsible for the observed increases in prevalence. He argues that there is a convergence of evidence about an abundance of studies, methods and multiple informants—with such increases being noticeable in all areas. It is also not to be expected that a similar trend towards openness to psychological symptoms could be observed in all countries of the globe. The fact that emotional and behavioral problems appear more frequently, but that the symptom of hyperactivity does not appear to change in frequency since years suggests that it may not be solely the sensitivity of parents or the openness of the societies which provide the main reasons for an increase in the prevalence of psychiatric symptoms and risk behaviors.

A second argument for the ostensible increase in mental health problems lies in the redefinition of mental disorders, as was done, for example, by the Diagnostic and Statistical Manual of Psychological Disorders DSM-5 [74]. Depending on the definition of the inclusion criteria, time criteria and intensity criteria, lower or higher prevalence numbers can be found. The introduction of "new" disorders in the DSM-5 can also change the overall prevalence of mental disorders: For example, intermittent explosive disorders, gender dysphoria, sleep-wake disorders, bipolar disorders or attenuated psychosis syndrome as a condition for further study are defined as clinical pictures in a uniqueness and in levels of details, like it has not been subjected to the diagnostic process before. If these diagnostic criteria are applied in addition to the classical diagnoses, this procedure can lead to an increase in the overall prevalence of mental problems. It must therefore always be kept in mind that there is a direct correlation between the definitions of mental disorders and the frequency of their occurrence. According to Collishaw [45], however, the argument of the "new definitions" of disorders alone is not able to satisfactorily explain the increasing prevalence numbers over the past 30 years, especially since these are represented in already known diagnostic groups like depression.

A third argument for the ostensible worldwide increase in mental disorders is the argument that normal psychological problems may be medicalized and subjected to psychiatric diagnoses. It is not uncommon for children in poverty or hostile environments to show physiological reactions to a pathological environment [35]. The children and adolescents who fear for their lives as unaccompanied refugees on the world's oceans, who grow up in war zones or are exposed to terrorist regimes, must not cynically be defined in their reactions as youngsters presenting with mental health problems! It would be scornful to diagnose disorders claiming a genetic weakness or vulnerability for them. However, their suffering must not be overlooked! The nosological description of psychological problems in adolescents under extreme conditions does not essentially address their problem. Psychological therapy should not be a fig leaf for social grievances, in these cases. Youngsters need empathy, solidarity and social support in their emergency situation. However, these arguments in no way explain why children in developed countries have increased mental health problems!

There are another three arguments for a real increase in psychological problems in childhood and adolescence: Many studies find increasing problem scores over time and refer to increased symptom rates rather than increased particular diagnoses [243]. An argument for the phenomenon that the global prevalence of mental disorders does not appear to be increasing as the prevalence increases at a young age could be that the onset of symptoms has shifted to earlier ages in recent decades. It could be that mental disorders nowadays already start in childhood and adolescence, which previously only appeared in adulthood. Long-term studies over the next few decades will show whether the actual increasing prevalence numbers among children and adolescents will eventually lead to an increase in the overall prevalence in adulthood, or whether they only indicate a shift in the onset of symptoms into the first two decades of life.

A second argument is social stratification. It can be clearly demonstrated that poverty and socio-economic deficiencies directly influence the extent of mental health problems in children and adolescents. The emotional problems for children from low- and middle-income families compared to children from high income families have increased fourfold in the last 25 years of the twentieth century! [45]. The Bella study also shows significant social influences on the frequency of symptoms over the course of the 6 years. Children with low socioeconomic status were overrepresented in the groups with recurrent or persistent symptoms compared to children with higher socioeconomic status [239]. In countries where the social gap between rich and poor continues to widen, the psychological problems in children and adolescents should also increase. The consequences of social adversities on the development of young people cannot be overestimated! The lifelong effects of early childhood adversities and toxic stress have implications for the practice of medicine, because it may be suggested that many adult diseases should be viewed as developmental phenomena that began in early life. Health disparities and risk behaviors or distorted life-styles are associated with poverty, discrimination or maltreatment and could be reduced or relieved and changed by the alleviation of toxic stress in childhood and adolescence [158].

The third argument concerns the possible increase in individual vulnerabilities. Some individuals may be more prone to particular symptoms or behaviors than others. The range of risk factors for physical and psychological development has changed significantly in recent decades. Due to the great advances in medicine, children with cancer or other pediatric systemic diseases can today be cured and survive in a very high percentage. The rate of premature babies that can survive today has also increased significantly. Do such children show higher rates of risk behavior in adolescence? No! Studies of adolescents who have had cancer show that they have lower rates of risk behaviors (such as smoking, alcohol or substance abuse) [244]. A follow-up examination of children with extremely low birth weight shows that these individuals had significantly fewer alcohol and substance abuse problems in young adulthood, but had an increased risk of other mental problems. Increased rates of anxiety disorders, social phobias or attention hyperactivity syndromes have been reported [245].

Another clue for changes in individual vulnerability could be the shift of the onset of puberty to earlier ages, since there is evidence that an earlier onset of puberty is associated with an increased risk of mental problems [45]. A meta-analysis has also shown that the amount of sleep in schoolchildren and adolescents has decreased significantly over the past 100 years [246]. The influence of such somatic parameters and risk behaviors on the development of psychological problems remains to be elucidated [10, 45]. Different patterns of risk behaviors and symptoms may be detected in different individuals due to their developmental history. There is also an individual vulnerability of adolescents due to interaction problems with their parents in childhood. This will be discussed in the following.

Research in the field of child and adolescent psychiatry has focused on the discovery of individual vulnerability factors for risk behaviors and psychopathological symptoms in recent decades. Such vulnerability means that under the given social circumstances, an individual is more likely to psychologically decompensate than individuals who do not have this characteristic. Implicitly, it thereby is expressed that the development of mental disorders may be due to a particular vulnerability or sensitivity of the individual, for example by a failure of its neurobiological or neuroendocrine systems. Is this a continuation of old basic ideas of, for example, A. Adler [234] who propagated the concept of organ inferiority for the development of mental disorders? At a methodologically high level, attempts have repeatedly been made to postulate a gene-environment interaction which shows that patients with certain genetic constellations are more prone to decompensation under unfavorable living conditions than people without this genetic constellation in similar psycho-social circumstances (overview in [35]).

One example of a potential vulnerability-gene is the MAO gene. A functional polymorphism of this neurotransmitter-metabolizing enzyme monoamine oxidase A (MAO-A) showed a differentiating effect on the influence of maltreatment on development in children and adolescents. Those children who had the genotype that showed high activity of the MAO-A gene were less likely to develop antisocial behaviors under unfavorable developmental conditions than those children who showed low MAO-A activity. Children with low MAO-A activity developed significant anti-social behaviors under abuse conditions. This study by Caspi and others [185], which was published in Science, could be finally supplemented by another paper in 2009 [188], in which the authors had shown that the activity of the MAO-A gene could also moderate beneficial effects on children. The authors examined the functional polymorphism in the regulator gene of the MAO-A gene and were able to show that stressors in childhood could be reduced by positive parenting in those children who showed a low activity of the regulator region of the MAO-A gene [188]. One could conclude that certain genetic constellations in the interaction between genes and the environment may not just represent a vulnerability, but that such "vulnerability genes" should rather be understood as "plasticity genes" [35].

It could be a convincing developmental principle: those who appear to be resistant to unfavorable circumstances and injuries also appear to be less responsive to favorable educational conditions. In contrast, people who are highly reactive to injuries and unfavorable circumstances could also be more open to warmth, clarity, comfort and positive parenting. In this sense, the genetic readiness would be more or less an expression of the plastic formability and responsiveness to different environments! Unfortunately, these gene-environment interactions of the MAO-A gene could not be confirmed in a large prospective study [190]. The individual vulnerability factors have not yet been deciphered in detail.

Belsky and Pluess [247] have focused on concepts beyond the diathesis-stress model. They describe various models of environmental sensitivity in children. Sensitivity enables children to respond and adapt to the challenges and opportunities associated with particular environmental conditions [248]. Individual differences in environmental sensitivity can be described. Differences in how people approach, respond, and interact with their immediate environment are reflected in psychological concepts like temperament or personality [248]. A growing number of empirical studies provide evidence for a predictive effect of temperament on environmental sensitivity [249]. The significant and distinctive contribution of new frameworks for the explanation of individual diatheses is the notion that sensitive individuals differ not only in their response to environmental adversity (e.g. child maltreatment)—as the traditional vulnerability concept implies—but also in response to positive supportive aspects of the environment (e.g. social support). This new aspect of variability in sensitivity to positive experiences is named vantage sensitivity [248]. These concepts may be integrated in models of environmental sensitivity with "vulnerability" as diathesis to stress, "resilience" as stress-resistance, "vantage sensitivity" as particular benefit from positive developmental influences and "vantage resistance" as a "blindness" to social support. The integrated concept can be read up in Pluess et al. [248]. There may be different individual constellations of all four sensitivity options. A growing number of empirical studies provide evidence that some children may be more affected by the quality of their environment than others [250]. Studies with the "highly sensitive child-scale" in 3581 children and adolescents suggest that there are three distinct groups of environmental sensitivity: low (25–35%), medium (41–47%) and high (20–35%). The high sensitivity group comprises the most important group of youngsters that may respond with symptoms to adversities and could benefit from social helping systems to the maximum.

10.3 Emotional Dialogue and Caregivers: The Family

As we have learned in Chap. 3 the emotional dialogue between mother and child plays a fundamental role in self-regulation of later developmental steps. The emotional expressions of the person in facial expressions, gestures and voice are understandable, quasi legible, and form the basis of the emotional dialogue, which—long before the child learns to speak—forms the interpersonal relationship between mother and child. Facial communication has a signal effect that can be used in relationship regulation [141]. Children have different abilities to deal with intense feelings from birth. This is operationalized in the temperament concepts. It seems that the basis of emotional regulation is a constitutional disposition—thought of as a temperament. From birth, children have different abilities to regulate their emotional states. However, this state regulation of the infant cannot be understood purely from a somatic point of view, because from the very beginning biological regulation is influenced by an interactional component of relationships with important caregivers [142]. Infants can be put into the emotional state in which their parents are by simply perceiving parental affects—such resonance phenomena have been repeatedly proven [30].

Even newborns react to the cries of other newborns with crying. We can call such phenomena emotional contagion [30]. Imitation affects can have both calming and disturbing effects in the child. In this way, facial expressions of the parents can not only reflect their own emotional state in a direct manner, but parents can also symbolically reflect thoughts and inner objects in their facial expressions when dealing with the child. This is also known as "as if communication". In this way, facial expressions can pass on information to the other person that goes beyond one's own state of affairs and convey and make available to others their own feelings (see Chap. 3). For example, caregivers can reflect the child's emotional state in their own facial expressions, in order to symbolically convey the child's emotions. This process is called emotional feedback. A phenomenon originally described by Gergely and Watson was finally conceptualized further by Fonagy in collaboration with the authors mentioned [144].

It appears that although the infant can already clearly show emotion expressions such as joy and grief, it does not yet have a clear awareness of the associated emotional states. The vague sensation of the inner states is ultimately brought to increasing awareness through the interaction with the important caregivers. In this way, parents can accentuate the utterances of the baby and, through playful forms with the children, influence the affects in the sense of co-regulation [30]. If, for example, a short smile on the child's face is deliberately grasped and mimed by the parents in such a way that the infant becomes aware of their own condition, the process of socio-emotional biofeedback is started. The infant recognizes that information about his own facial expressions, his own emotional state is reflected, which he can use to increase awareness of his own. This is only possible through a specific marking in the caregiver's expressions of emotion, a marking that indicates that the affect shown by the parents applies to the child himself.

Another interactive mechanism has a significant impact on affect regulation and the development of meaning in the child. It is "social referencing" (according to [146]). Social referencing refers to the tendency of the toddler to face the mother when confronted with interesting or unsettling objects and to adapt his own reactions to her facial expression and voice. If the mother communicates an anxiety affect, the child may have an anxious reaction, but if she smiles reassuringly, the child can continue to show curiosity. Such social referencing processes can be used to communicate affective evaluations and share them between the caregiver and the child. In this way, the child's emotional responsiveness can be influenced favorably. The child is not only exposed to an unsettling environment, but can constitute meanings in dialogue with the caregiver (see Chap. 3).

These emotional biofeedback-related regulations of the child and their interactive procedural design will be supplemented in later ages by symbolic exchange processes using gestures, words, and narratives between the caregiver and the child. It can be assumed that deficiencies in the early phase of interactively reflecting emotional regulation can continue later in impairments of the symbolic exchange processes [142].

It follows from the above that disturbances in the emotional dialogue, for example, due to the psychological impairment of the parents, can lead to an unfavorable development of the child's emotional regulation. According to Plass & Wiegand-Grefe [251], a three to seven times higher psychological abnormality rate was found in children of parents with psychiatric illness compared to the total population. It can be assumed that around 500,000 children in Germany grow up with a depressed parent. In a long-term study in children of depressed parents over a period of 20 years, depressive disorders were found in 21% of the offspring compared to 8% in a control group (review by [251]). The risk of depression is tripled in children of depressed parents! A meta-analysis of 25 studies on offspring of parents with anxiety disorders reveals that when parents had an anxiety disorder than the offspring were significantly more likely to have anxiety (risk ratio 1.76) and depressive disorder (risk ratio 1.31) compared to offspring of parents without anxiety disorders [252]. Parental psychiatric symptoms do have a negative effect on the outcome of children's psychopathology. A study aimed at monitoring internalizing and externalizing symptoms in 742 mothers, 440 fathers and their 811 children in 3 outpatient clinics. 1.7 years later a follow up was done. Higher symptom scores at follow up were found in those children whose mothers or fathers scored above the subclinical threshold for psychiatric symptoms at baseline. Children of parents with psychiatric symptoms are at risk for persisting symptoms themselves [253]. To explore whether paternal psychological distress is related to the longitudinal course of child problem behavior after accounting for maternal psychological distress the following study was designed. Data were taken from the Millenium Cohort Study in United Kingdom and analyzed using growth curve modeling in 13,442 individuals. There was evidence for a robust association between psychological distress in fathers and problem behavior in their offspring. It is suggested, that the mental health of both mothers and fathers are important for the behavior of their children [254].

Children of mentally ill parents are subject to destructive parentification [251]. Parents give up their parental function and abuse the child in the sense of satisfying their own needs. The child's needs are clearly neglected. The child is pushed into a developmental role that is not suitable for children, which can ultimately also cross generations. The child must assume a responsibility that is not appropriate for its age and its stage of development and must subordinate its own needs to the requirements set by the parents. Furthermore, the child does not receive adequate recognition for taking on these special tasks (lack of reciprocity of giving and taking,

[251]). In children of mentally ill parents, the destructive emotional impact of a lack of parental function is evident. But could a subtle disruption of the emotional dialogue lead to problems even under less severe impairments of the parental function? In a meta-analysis, the composition of families in the sense of new patchwork constellations with different distribution of responsibility does not seem to have a primary effect on unfavorable mental health trends [45]. Connections with general trends in social development will be discussed in the following.

Child maltreatment of all types is a serious concern for society. A German study compared datasets of two population based nationwide surveys in 2010 and 2016 in both instances with more than 2500 participants aged 14 years and older, who had been selected randomly. Information about childhood experiences was obtained. Maltreatment seemed to slightly decrease from 35.3% in 2010 to 31.0% in 2016. However, the percentages of adolescents who reported multiple types of maltreatment remained stable over the years. The study concludes, that the systems in place for monitoring the occurrence of child maltreatment in Germany are insufficient at present [255].

10.4 Education and School

The school is repeatedly attributed to a negative function for the development of children. Increasing pressure to perform is blamed for "burnout problems in children" [256]. On closer inspection, however, school often turns out to be a resource for children, especially when they have to live in difficult domestic conditions. It does not seem to be so much the requirement for performance that puts children under pressure—children are naturally keen to perform and want to exercise and develop themselves. Rather, it seems to be the pressure to succeed—to always be the best in comparison with the others—that makes life difficult for children. If all children in a class are required to be among the best in the class in order to be successful later, this can only lead to a demotivation and humiliation of the majority. We should therefore focus more on the uncritical pressure to succeed that the over-ambitious adults give the children and adolescents. The aim of education should be culture and not competition.

The behavior of young people towards each other in the area of school can also influence the risk of mental problems or induce risk behaviors with school absence or school refusal (see Chap. 2). Bullying in schools has become the focus of public and academic attention in recent years [123]. The harassment, bullying and torture that children share with each other can also be extended to the areas of new media and the internet in the sense of cyberbullying. It is characteristic of the bullying that it makes other children and adolescents to victims who cannot defend themselves against the accusations in the given situation. Prevalence figures show that around 13% of school students surveyed can be affected as victims, 11% as perpetrators and 4% as victims and perpetrators [123]. In our own investigation, we were able to make it clear that the pressure of suffering from school bullying is enormous and that the risk of emotional disorders and behavioral problems is increased on both the victim and the perpetrator side. School careers can also be significantly affected. In our own study, 20.8% of students said they had been victim of bullying in the past few months. The risk of developing emotional disorders such as depression, suicidality and self-harming behaviors was significantly increased for victimized students. Risks for these emotional problems and risk behaviors were found to increase 2.4 to threefold [123]. From these results, the needs to drive the expansion of school-related bullying prevention programs in Europe can be derived. It is believed that preventing school bullying can actually help reduce risk behaviors and serious emotional disorders in adolescents.

If you look at the trends of the economic development in the countries of Europe, you will notice dramatically high youth unemployment, especially in southern countries [257]. If the educational career of children and adolescents stagnates at the transition to social responsibility, this clearly has an unfavorable impact on the development conditions for children and adolescents. Children need development, education and career opportunities to stay mentally healthy. Anyone who learns at an early age that society will not provide chances for the future will have to wither and fail due to psychological stress factors. The current crisis with coronavirus disease (COVID-19) will make the situation even more complicated. It can be assumed that the economic situation in several European countries will worsen, which will have a particularly negative impact on unemployment among young people. The problem of poverty and lack of prospects will tend not to become smaller, but larger.

There are substantial health disparities between children from low- and higher-income families [258]. Substantiated differences could be assessed in parent and teacher reported symptom scores in 11-year-old children of three waves of the Child and Adolescent Mental Health Survey and the Millenium Cohort Study. Marked child mental health inequalities do exist. The mental health gap between advantaged and disadvantaged children has not reduced over the last 20 years and may even be getting worse [258]. To provide opportunities for development and participation may be more important than psychiatric interventions in the first line.

10.5   Zeitgeist: The Seven Plagues

Our civilization of a high-tech and globally oriented society has repeatedly been used socio-philosophically with the term "postmodern" to express that we have left an era of modern change in traditional structures behind [259]. The term postmodernity was coined by Jean-Francois Lyotard [260] and referred to a zeitgeist that is not characterized by a single direction, a style, a fashion, a myth and a binding history of a cultural epoch, but rather a social system that comprises diversity and ambiguity, while it is shaped by multi-values and multidimensionality of claims and expectations. The patchwork is a good picture for our present times [259]. A problem with this postmodern diversity is the confusion and arbitrariness of opinions, knowledge and attitudes [261]. Even if it seemed like a liberation from the shackles of expert's opinions and was to be considered from an emancipatory point of view, to question our tools of cognition and knowledge and to give more weight to the different subjective considerations of the individual, this "primacy of interpretations over the facts" brought us new painful experiences. It was a fallacy of postmodernism that any form of knowledge could be an instrument of submission and that skepticism towards the reality as such already has an emancipatory power [262]. Because relativism has played into the hands of more and more cynical demagogues in recent years, who eventually served people's wishful thinking through propaganda, while mercilessly pursuing neoliberal and authoritarian or religious interests that favored a small elite at the expense of most of society [261]. In a world of terror, warmongering, cold capitalism, and internal European tensions, after stock market crises and the bursting of the economic bubble, we see the general conditions of our life differently today. Today there are realities that cannot be overlooked, disasters that deal with life and death and that touch upon existence—that are not just mind games [261]. It is therefore also important to recognize the neo-realistic principle, the realities, in our postmodern information society. It is obviously not true that only subjective realities and interpretations prevail over what we call reality. There are things that are not to be trifled with, that cannot be interpreted away and that do not disappear through words and that are not expressions of mere opinion: facts such as death, trauma, loneliness, pain, or poverty [261]. The coronavirus (COVID-19) pandemic has painfully taught us that recently.

Even in the center of Europe—in our affluent society—despite welfare, technical excellence, a wealth of information, and opportunities for development, we must not ignore the breaks in continuity, the breaks in tradition and the movement of values, the misrepresentation and acceleration of adaptation of the present [35].

The question must be asked, at what degree of multiplication of possibilities does the arbitrariness begin? When do breaks and new beginnings lead to dismemberment and when acceleration becomes madness? The zenith of feasibility has been reached in many fields; nanotechnology, genetic engineering and computer technology have led to continental shifts in social processes and in the value discussions that have permeated everyday family life, the service sector, and the educational landscape. The change in social structures with radical economic principles opens up new horizons of meaning for the previous basic concepts of human relationship and education culture [259]. At what point in time of flexible social guidelines does a chaos of orientation begin in the subjective experience of the individual? When can diversity finally become weary? Byung-Chul Han [263] shows how the abundance of choices can lead to stiffness, paralysis or numbness and how self-exploitation ultimately leads to excessive demands. Our present is thus determined by a polarity between the agony of choice and the opportunities to act. Critical valuation and meaning are required. In their article, Resch and Westhoff [259] highlighted seven important points that undermine the adaptation efforts of the adolescents in the present:

- *Variety of information.* Our time is characterized by an unprecedented variety of information. The internet provides access to world knowledge from art treasures to instructions for making bombs. Worldwide news services overwhelm us with a flood of images, which can lead to sensory overload if there is a lack of selection or which fixes the individual in an addictive spell in the fleeting access to images. The valuable and the cheap are offered to the consumer on an equal footing. Development-endangering and enriching things have to be filtered and assessed by the consumer himself.

- *Success orientation.* Competitive pressure and a focus on success lead to the necessary processes of lifelong learning and effort. The work process requires all employees to be guided by performance criteria, perfected guidelines and a benchmarking system that increasingly encourages the economization of everyday life. But it is not enough to solve a (self) task, to penetrate a problem, to achieve a goal: Again and again it is demanded to be better than others, being among the winners, to replace the best with even better things. Everyday life is an all-round competition.
- *Complexity of social problems.* The social situation has become so complex that it results in an unmanageability of social phenomena for many. Rarely do causal models make a lasting statement. Politics are based on expertise, but it is not uncommon for them to have contradictory recommendations. Experts often provide contradictory interpretations of the same data. In the area of the economic system, in particular, ideologies are misunderstood as scientific models. There are also no simple solutions in a globalized world in climate issues, refugee policy, and military-strategic decisions. Many decisions, especially in the political field, have to be made from a system perspective and cybernetic rule laws. Even those who poke in the fog still have to act prudently, while a worried mob takes to the streets in dull slogans.
- *Diversity of values.* In a globalized world, a variety of values of religious, economic and aesthetic judgments have emerged. This causes the seeker to be uncertain about what is right and what is wrong. There is no guideline, no uniqueness in questions of values.
- *Cultural diversity.* The cultural diversity and intersection of different ethnic groups enables interesting encounters on the one hand, but also harbors the dangers of clashing different cultures [264]. Usually, those who fear the unknown tend to escape to fundamentalist and xenophobic concepts.
- *Mobility.* The mobility demanded by globalization encourages family separation in countries with good economic conditions. It is important for employees to forego settling down and being rooted in their own careers. This contrasts with the need for ties and relationships in the microsystem of the family. It is becoming increasingly difficult to define a place to be at home. Due to the increasing burden of war and terror, on the other hand, huge flows of refugees have made their way to ensure their survival. The fortress Europe will not be able to assert itself in xenophobic isolation as an island of the blessed without betraying its central values and ideals.
- *Flexibility and change of social roles.* Flexibility of thinking, changeability of social roles and different spheres of life are required of the individual on his development path. Changing jobs, changing roles and changing locations

increasingly creates the risk of arbitrariness and social diffusion. The profiles of the work have changed through new technologies and the influence of the new information media. Artificial intelligence replaces humans. Automated production chains rarefy job opportunities; less well-trained workers have to worry about their jobs. The corona crisis has even exacerbated these problems.

In this described field of tension, the adolescents have to achieve their personal identity, a solid self-image and a stable self-worth. The postmodern opportunities and the dangers addressed in the new realism require a high quality of education and training, a high level of self-reflection and self-control, as well as good emotional differentiation with communicative competence of the individual [265]. While some authors interpret the social impact on family systems as "not so bad" (e. g. [266]), other authors speak of social acceleration [43] and breeding grounds of uncertainty [267]. Byung-Chul Han [268] even goes so far in his book that he speaks of self-exploitation of the fatigue society. In the abundance of what is possible [269] and in the hamster wheel of narcissistic self-exploitation [270], we have seen a change in the conditions for the failure of particular individuals. Today it is suggested to the young person that all chances are open, but this offer of being able to achieve everything is not true! If everything were supposed to be attainable, then failure and the restrictions that the individual experiences remain attached to the individual himself. The less self-esteem, security of identity and expectation of success the individual brings with it, the more he stabilizes himself in this uncertainty of decision with risk behavior [259]. Whereas in the past the prevailing narrowing of a neurotic superstructure was the motto "I must not" and gave rise to feelings of guilt and narrowing the scope for action, today "I am not allowed to" has given way to an excess of a sobering and humiliating "I cannot" [259]. If you have the feeling of inferiority, convinced that you can't do it, you can't bring it, self-contempt has reached its peak. Shame is the central emotion.

10.6 Threatened Emotional Dialogue

Given these framework conditions of an increasingly globalized present—with critical narrowing of individual recovery phases, diversity of chances and dangers of temptation—do they influence the emotional dialogue in the dyad between caregivers and children? Don't the adults, annoyed and exhausted by the increased stress of everyday life and their own disorientation, refrain from the emotional dialogue with their children? [259] Isn't there a lack of time, causing impatience, misunderstanding and a lack of fit—up to neglect and psychological traumatization—in the parent-child interactions? Under conditions in which the adults themselves already have psychological disorders, children are forced into early independence and exposed to dysfunctional parenting influences. Another mechanism applies to parents who do narcissistically charge the children. These parents themselves are set under time pressure and pressure to succeed. Their children become the focus of families, but not according to their needs, but rather as a source of hope and human capital, which is put under special focus to succeed and praised for the smallest learning steps. Children are pampered and challenged at the same time. Attention and affection are linked to performance requirements. Small everyday problems are cleared out of the way. Children develop the illusion of being able to control their surroundings. However, if they do not reach the required goal, they are afraid of being dropped. Small everyday problems then become stumbling blocks that seem insurmountable. Avoidance and withdrawal may result.

Anyway, adolescents often remain materially dependent on their parents for many years and additionally become socially and mentally dependent. The combination of disorientation of the adolescent with pampering care from the parents is hostile to development [18]. While children are charged with narcissism in their significance, primarily fulfilling parents' wishes is a risk factor for narcissistic self-development [259]. There are several ways to fail, but many of them lead through the topic of mutual not being "good enough" and not being able to decide [35].

There is an increasing gap between the requirements for adaptation to societal demands for our young people and the increasing social and emotional problems in the families. We have to assume that the impairment of the emotional interplay in the microsystem due to the diverse factors of social influences (job insecurity, time pressure, media overstimulation and exhaustion) on the caregivers can ultimately weaken the child's personality development. A disrupted emotional dialogue with the important caregivers may have a negative impact on the self-regulation of the offspring (see Fig. 10.1). Single parents do have a special risk of not meeting children's needs by loneliness and exhaustion. Parents with psychiatric disturbances are particularly at risk of making relationships with their children dysfunctional. Taking into account the three tenets of resilience [139] important developmental milestones of plasticity, sociability, and meaning cannot be evolved. On the basis of a disrupted development of psychic structure and self-regulation, adolescents are less and less willing and able to meet the challenges of everyday life in society. If adolescents develop mental problems and difficulties arise in the process of identity

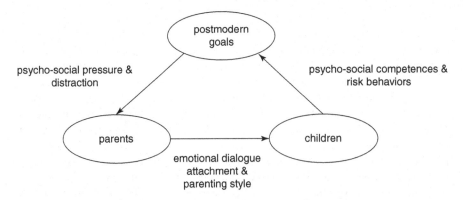

Fig. 10.1 The developmental triangle of risk behavior

development, self-esteem regulation, intimacy, and social role development in adolescent years, risk behaviors and the non-fulfillment of adolescent development tasks must result from these facts. There would then be an increased consumption of leisure time, media, alcohol, and drugs. These consumer behaviors work like crutches for the adolescents, they provide a substitute world [259].

Others aggressively vent their displeasure and lack of opportunities. The "no future attitude" and the learned helplessness, just like the so-called "burn-out syndrome" [256], are only other formulations for depressive developments. After all, the internalized accusation of being inadequate, the self-blaming for one's own failure and the hopelessness on the threshold of growing up cannot ultimately remain without consequences. And where young people endanger themselves in their development through risk behaviors, they get into a vicious cycle of self-harm up to suicide attempts and they fail to reach adult levels in their identity-diffusion, shame and self-doubt [35].

10.7 Helper Systems and Psychotherapy

What could the shift of psychological stress and irritation to younger and younger ages of our offspring have to do with ourselves as parents or as professional helpers? Are we the appropriate role models and figures of identification, do we offer the right relationship contexts? Do we support the emotional development of the personalities of our children and adolescents through commitment, respect, and reliable rituals providing the appreciation of the other as an equal human being [259]? The overwhelmed individual returns from his social explorations in the haze of today's social developments as a victim or potential perpetrator with destructive potential. And in all self-injuries and escalating risk behaviors, the young people make it clear to themselves and others that they are only material, that they have only become worthless "things", objects on which desperate activities are lived out [259]. In such a paradox of self-reification and addiction-like self-consumption, the longing to assert oneself and to define something of one's own is finally staged. This paradox can only be resolved by us adults in the sense of differentiated intersubjectivity. This is one of the greatest tasks for the future for all of us [35]. The corona-pandemic opens up a new chapter in the book of adversities. We still do not know how the economic and social consequences will shape the development of our next generations. However, it can be taken for granted that the problems of micro-system erosion and the disruption of the emotional dialogue between parents and their offspring will continue to impinge on coherence of adolescent's selves.

Does psychotherapy help the threatened individuals? Psychotherapy moves in a field of tension between emancipatory demands on the one hand and the desire to optimize psychological functions on the other. A dialectical movement can be determined. The aspect of freedom—as the basic idea of psychotherapy—cannot be emphasized enough. The goal must be to bring about increased degrees of freedom for adolescents. The optimization of the psychic inner world by changing neuronal functions must be thoroughly reflected as a therapeutic goal, because such an improvement indeed may increase the degrees of freedom of the individual concerned, but ultimately subjects the patient to the ideas and attitudes of the therapist. We believe that we give the depressed person more freedom by changing the biological conditions of the restrictive depression—a disorder, which reduces or even prohibits the patient's freedom. An attempt is made to establish the basis for the greatest possible psychological flexibility in the individual [271]. However, we do not escape the problem that we as psychotherapists want to use both elements of neuro-enhancement and emancipation therapeutically! It remains important that the patient himself agrees with the external goals of change and improvement. It is not about us therapists believing that we know a little better what is "actually" good for the patient or would benefit him, and then impose this idea on the patient. That would be mere neuro-pedagogy and optimizing brain functions alone is no help. It is much more important to achieve joint movement in the intersubjective field with the patient. The intersubjective field cannot be determined by one of the participants alone, it is the result of a successful coordination, more a mental resonance [272] than a cognitive construction. Exaggerated self-protection, defense, or the egocentrism of the individual involved disrupt the intersubjective field. It's more about hitting or missing a common frequency. It's about inclinations and attitudes, not just explanations and knowledge transfer. Only self-realized knowledge (learning by heart) can help change such attitudes. In any case, mutual recognition and respect are central requirements of the intersubjective field. Such considerations are in the tradition of Donna Orange et al. [273] and Stolorow et al. [274].

The tension between emancipation and neuro-enhancement can be described as follows [275]: From an emancipatory point of view, the soul has a neuronal basis, but its demands and effects go far beyond that. From a neurobiological point of view, the soul is merely an epiphenomenon of neuronal functions. From the point of view of emancipation, the patient's internal goals are revealed, detected and promoted, thus the patient is offered help for self-help. From the point of view of enhancement, external goals are made achievable by optimizing neuronal functions. The patient only has the freedom to make decisions to participate or not, the choice of destination is taken away. While emancipatory endeavors enable liberation and unleashing of people, there is a risk of manipulation and external control in enhancement, which can result in external determination. In contrast, the promotion of self-determination is open to the polyvalence of the goals that a patient strives for in self-authorship, whereby we as therapists offer support in the intersubjective field. From the point of view of enhancement, a goal chosen by the therapist must be focused, which the patient tries to achieve in a success-oriented manner. The danger here is further self-exploitation of personal resources. Psychotherapy always moves within this bi-polar field between enhancement and emancipation in a dialectical manner, whereby artistic and creative therapy methods can expand the intersubjective field in the direction of emancipation.

Psychotherapy may help individuals who present with risk behaviors and threaten their future chances. Psychotherapy is not a substitute for religion and not a lifestyle drug. Psychotherapy cannot compensate for a lack of standard of living and a lack of meaning in everyday life through professional interventions [261]. It is also not intended to support self-staging and ego design or to compensate for the spiritual deficits of disappointed egomaniacs. Psychotherapy is a method of treating sick and suffering people and is not designed to meet overexcited demands from parents against their children and adolescents.

It is important to explore the inner values and potentials of psychotherapy. In which way and how can psychotherapy activate resources and initiate emancipatory processes?

We summarize: The skepticism towards the attempts to economically restrict psychotherapy and to devalue it in favor of somatic or pharmacological therapy measures, to trivialize it and to misuse it as a substitute for religion must not go so far that we throw the child out with the bath-water and understand psychotherapy as a "scientifically suspicious" therapy measure. Psychotherapy has a sound method and a humanitarian concern. Both represent an empirical and a philosophical reality.

We must not forget that self-discovery is always a piece of self-invention! But what we must equally not forget is that each self also has a real and potentially destructible core part in its mere interpersonal presence. This appreciation for each other's self is the starting point for psychotherapeutic work.

Chapter 11
Take Home Messages

The book is based on the idea that epidemiologically increasing juvenile risk behaviors—like substance abuse, non-suicidal self-injury (NSSI), antisocial or suicidal behavior—serve the adolescent's self to fulfill developmental tasks like identity-formation and regulation of self-worth. Three questions are addressed:

What?—what are the developmental problems of young people like? What are the developmental tasks to be fulfilled during adolescence? What is the purpose of risk behaviors in the everyday life of emergent adulthood? What symptoms do adolescents increasingly suffer from?

How?—how can risk behaviors be thoroughly diagnosed in the nosological framework? How can these symptoms be interpreted contextually? How can the personal structure of the self be understood? How does the cybernetic view on symptoms change our therapeutic view? How can the influence of cybernetics on psychopathology be understood? How can risk behaviors be interpreted in the light of cybernetic principles of the "Perceptual Control Theory"? How can a functional symptom analysis be performed step by step? How can symptoms be understood based on functional contextualism?

Why?—Why does new morbidity present with an increase in symptom prevalence? Why do we find differential susceptibility to environmental influences? Why does the disruption of the emotional dialogue in parent child-interaction change the adolescent's chances to participate in social domains?

The threat of the acceleration of social processes, the risks of postmodern society will be considered. Narcissistic self-exploitation, mobility tasks, flexibility and the challenges of new media perform a social pressure on parental figures, distract and overstrain their mental resources thus changing and dissolving the emotional dialogue with their children. Children themselves experience a neglect and impoverishment of emotional bonding—resulting in a lack of self-regulating capacities in adolescence. Risk behaviors are the consequences. Help can only be offered, if there

F. Resch, P. Parzer, *Adolescent Risk Behavior and Self-Regulation*, https://doi.org/10.1007/978-3-030-69955-0_11

is an understanding of the adaptive functions of risk behaviors and symptoms. Risk behaviors may represent precursors of more serious mental disorders, and in the worst case can also turn into those disorders of a disease nature. However, the starting point is always the lifestyle-behavior, triggered by environmental circumstances in the light of individual goals.

References

1. Kessler RC, Berglund P, Demler O, et al. Lifetime prevalence and age-of-onset distributions of DSM-IV disorders in the National Comorbidity Survey Replication. Arch Gen Psychiatry. 2005;62:593–602. https://doi.org/10.1001/archpsyc.62.6.593.
2. Kaess M, Brunner R, Parzer P, et al. Risk-behaviour screening for identifying adolescents with mental health problems in Europe. Eur Child Adolesc Psychiatry. 2014;23:611–20. https://doi.org/10.1007/s00787-013-0490-y.
3. Polanczyk GV, Salum GA, Sugaya LS, et al. Annual research review: a meta-analysis of the worldwide prevalence of mental disorders in children and adolescents. J Child Psychol Psychiatry. 2015;56:345–65. https://doi.org/10.1111/jcpp.12381.
4. Walker EF, Sabuwalla Z, Huot R. Pubertal neuromaturation, stress sensitivity, and psychopathology. Dev Psychopathol. 2004;16:807–24. https://doi.org/10.1017/s0954579404040027.
5. Giedd JN. Structural magnetic resonance imaging of the adolescent brain. Ann N Y Acad Sci. 2004;1021:77–85. https://doi.org/10.1196/annals.1308.009.
6. Casey BJ, Jones RM, Hare TA. The adolescent brain. Ann N Y Acad Sci. 2008;1124:111–26. https://doi.org/10.1196/annals.1440.010.
7. Konrad K, Firk C, Uhlhaas PJ. Hirnentwicklung in der Adoleszenz: Neurowissenschaftliche Befunde zum Verständnis dieser Entwicklungsphase. Dtsch Arztebl Int. 2013;110:425–31. https://doi.org/10.3238/arztebl.2013.0425.
8. Maslowsky J, Owotomo O, Huntley ED, Keating D. Adolescent risk behavior: differentiating reasoned and reactive risk-taking. J Youth Adolesc. 2019;48:243–55. https://doi.org/10.1007/s10964-018-0978-3.
9. Whittle S, Dennison M, Vijayakumar N, et al. Childhood maltreatment and psychopathology affect brain development during adolescence. J Am Acad Child Adolesc Psychiatry. 2013;52:940–952.e1. https://doi.org/10.1016/j.jaac.2013.06.007.
10. Short MA, Weber N. Sleep duration and risk-taking in adolescents: a systematic review and meta-analysis. Sleep Med Rev. 2018;41:185–96. https://doi.org/10.1016/j.smrv.2018.03.006.
11. Fecteau S, Knoch D, Fregni F, et al. Diminishing risk-taking behavior by modulating activity in the prefrontal cortex: a direct current stimulation study. J Neurosci. 2007;27:12500–5. https://doi.org/10.1523/JNEUROSCI.3283-07.2007.
12. Resch F, Lehmkuhl G. Adoleszenz—junges Erwachsenenalter: Entwicklungsdynamik und Entwicklungsaufgaben. In: Lehmkuhl G, Resch F, Herpertz SC, editors. Psychotherapie des jungen Erwachsenenalters: Basiswissen für die Praxis und störungsspezifische Behandlungsansätze. Stuttgart: Kohlhammer; 2015. p. 17–26.
13. Kutscher N. Jugend und Medien. In: Rauschenbach T, Borrmann S, editors. Herausforderungen des Jugendalters. Weinheim: Beltz Juventa; 2013. p. 118–38.

14. Nesi J, Choukas-Bradley S, Prinstein MJ. Transformation of adolescent peer relations in the social media context. Part 1—a theoretical framework and application to dyadic peer relationships. Clin Child Fam Psychol Rev. 2018;21:267–94. https://doi.org/10.1007/s10567-018-0261-x.
15. Spitzer M. Digitale Demenz: wie wir uns und unsere Kinder um den Verstand bringen. München: Droemer; 2014.
16. Resch F, Kaess M. Risikoverhalten bei Jugendlichen. Ruperto Carola Forschungsmagazin. 2017;11:61–7.
17. Arnett JJ. Emerging adulthood: the winding road from the late teens through the twenties. Oxford: Oxford University Press; 2004.
18. Seiffge-Krenke I. Therapieziel Identität: Veränderte Beziehungen, Krankheitsbilder und Therapie. Stuttgart: Klett-Cotta; 2012.
19. Resch F, Sevecke K. Identität—Eine Illusion? Selbstentwicklung in der Adoleszenz. Prax Kinderpsychol Kinderpsychiatr. 2018;67:613–23. https://doi.org/10.13109/prkk.2018.67.7.613.
20. Oerter R. Kultur, Ökologie und Entwicklung. In: Oerter R, Montada L, editors. Entwicklungspsychologie: ein Lehrbuch, 3. vollständig überarb. und erw. Weinheim: Aufl. Beltz; 1995. p. 84–127.
21. Wygotski LS. Denken und Sprechen. Berlin: Akad. Verl; 1964.
22. Resch F. Entwicklungspsychopathologie des Kindes- und Jugendalters. Weinheim: Psychologie Verlags Union; 1996.
23. Havighurst RJ. Developmental tasks and education. New York: McKay; 1972.
24. Freud A. The ego and the mechanisms of defence. London: Karnac Books; 1937.
25. Seiffge-Krenke I. Chronic disease and perceived developmental progression in adolescence. Dev Psychol. 1998;34:1073–84.
26. Böhme G. Ich-Selbst und der Andere. In: Liessmann KP, editor. Ich—der Einzelne in seinen Netzen. Wien: Zsolnay; 2014. p. 53–65.
27. Resch F. Identität und Ablösung—Entwicklungsaufgaben der Adoleszenz. Swiss Arch Neurol Psychiatr Psychother. 2016;167:137–46. https://doi.org/10.4414/sanp.2016.00411.
28. Scharfetter C. Allgemeine Psychopathologie. Stuttgart: Thieme; 1991.
29. Dornes M. Der kompetente Säugling. Frankfurt: Fischer; 1993.
30. Dornes M. Die Seele des Kindes: Entstehung und Entwicklung. Frankfurt: Fischer; 2006.
31. Newen A. Philosophie des Geistes: Eine Einführung. 1st ed. München: C. H. Beck; 2013.
32. Descombes V. Die Rätsel der Identität. Berlin: Suhrkamp; 2013.
33. Möhler E. Eltern-Säuglings-Psychotherapie. München: Reinhardt; 2013.
34. Taubner S, Volkert J. Mentalisierungs-Basierte Therapie für Adoleszente. Göttingen: Vandenhoeck & Ruprecht; 2017.
35. Resch F, Parzer P. Neue Morbidität und Zeitgeist. In: Brähler E, Herzog W, editors. Sozialpsychosomatik: Das vergessene Soziale in der Psychosomatischen Medizin. Stuttgart: Schattauer; 2018. p. 319–35.
36. Erikson EH. Identity and the life cycle: selected papers. New York: International Universities Press; 1959.
37. Marcia JE. Ego identity: a handbook for psychosocial research. New York: Springer; 1993.
38. Luyckx K, Schwartz SJ, Goossens L, et al. Processes of personal identity formation and evaluation. In: Schwartz SJ, Luyckx K, Vignoles VL, editors. Handbook of identity theory and research. New York: Springer; 2011. p. 77–98.
39. Kroger J, Martinussen M, Marcia JE. Identity status change during adolescence and young adulthood: a meta-analysis. J Adolesc. 2010;33:683–98. https://doi.org/10.1016/j.adolescence.2009.11.002.
40. Seiffge-Krenke I, Besevegis E, Chau C, et al. Identitätsentwicklung, Familienbeziehungen und Symptombelastung bei Jugendlichen aus sieben Ländern. Prax Kinderpsychol Kinderpsychiatr. 2018;67:639–56. https://doi.org/10.13109/prkk.2018.67.7.639.
41. Goth K, Foelsch P, Schlüter-Müller S, et al. Assessment of identity development and identity diffusion in adolescence—theoretical basis and psychometric properties of the self-report

questionnaire AIDA. Child Adolesc Psychiatry Ment Health. 2012;6:27. https://doi.org/10.118 6/1753-2000-6-27.

42. Seiffge-Krenke I. Die Jugendlichen und ihre Suche nach dem neuen Ich: Identitätsentwicklung in der Adoleszenz. Stuttgart: Kohlhammer; 2020.

43. Rosa H. Beschleunigung: die Veränderung der Zeitstrukturen in der Moderne. Frankfurt: Suhrkamp; 2005.

44. Sennett R. The corrosion of character: the personal consequences of work in the new capitalism. New York: Norton; 1998.

45. Collishaw S. Annual research review: secular trends in child and adolescent mental health. J Child Psychol Psychiatry. 2015;56:370–93. https://doi.org/10.1111/jcpp.12372.

46. Resch F, Möhler E. Entwicklungspsychologie des Narzissmus. In: Kernberg OF, Hartmann H-P, editors. Narzissmus: Grundlagen—Störungsbilder—Therapie. Stuttgart: Schattauer; 2006. p. 37–70.

47. Resch F, Romer G, Schmeck K, Seiffge-Krenke I, editors. OPD-CA-2 operationalized psychodynamic diagnosis in childhood and adolescence: theoretical basis and user manual. Göttingen: Hogrefe; 2017.

48. Erikson EH. Identity, youth, and crisis. New York: W. W Norton; 1968.

49. Resch F. Mr. L and his therapy process: a case discussion. psychoanalysis. Self Context. 2020;15:58–61. https://doi.org/10.1080/24720038.2019.1677670.

50. Winnicott DW. The theory of the parent-infant relationship. Int J Psychoanal. 1960;41: 585–95.

51. DiClemente RJ, Hansen WB, Ponton LE, editors. Handbook of adolescent health risk behavior. Berlin: Springer Science & Business Media; 1996.

52. Knollmann M, Reissner V, Hebebrand J. Towards a comprehensive assessment of school absenteeism: development and initial validation of the inventory of school attendance problems. Eur Child Adolesc Psychiatry. 2019;28:399–414. https://doi.org/10.1007/s00787-018-1204-2.

53. Lenzen C, Fischer G, Jentzsch A, et al. Schulabsentismus in Deutschland—Die Prävalenz von entschuldigten und unentschuldigten Fehlzeiten und ihre Korrelation mit emotionalen und Verhaltensauffälligkeiten. Prax Kinderpsychol Kinderpsychiatr. 2013;62:570–82.

54. du Bois R, Resch F, editors. Klinische Psychotherapie des Jugendalters: ein integratives Praxisbuch. Stuttgart: Kohlhammer; 2005.

55. Koenig J, Fischer-Waldschmidt G, Brunner R, et al. Zuflucht in digitalen Welten - zum Zusammenhang von kritischen Lebensereignissen mit pathologischem Internetgebrauch im Jugendalter. Prax Kinderpsychol Kinderpsychiatr. 2016;65:494–515. https://doi.org/10.13109/prkk.2016.65.7.494.

56. Resch F, du Bois R. Die Entwicklungspsychopathologie der Jugendkrisen. In: du Bois R, Resch F, editors. Klinische Psychotherapie des Jugendalters: ein integratives Praxisbuch. Stuttgart: Kohlhammer; 2005. p. 33–52.

57. Resch F, Parzer P. Entwicklungspsychopathologie und Psychotherapie: Kybernetische Modelle zur funktionellen Diagnostik bei Jugendlichen. Wiesbaden: Springer; 2015.

58. Kaess M, Edinger A. Selbstverletzendes Verhalten. 2nd ed. Weinheim: Beltz; 2019.

59. Firth J, Solmi M, Wootton RE, et al. A meta-review of "lifestyle psychiatry": the role of exercise, smoking, diet and sleep in the prevention and treatment of mental disorders. World Psychiatry. 2020;19:360–80. https://doi.org/10.1002/wps.20773.

60. Romer D, Reyna VF, Satterthwaite TD. Beyond stereotypes of adolescent risk taking: placing the adolescent brain in developmental context. Dev Cogn Neurosci. 2017;27:19–34. https://doi.org/10.1016/j.dcn.2017.07.007.

61. Igra V, Irwin CE. Theories of adolescent risk taking behavior. In: Di Clemente RJ, Hansen WB, Ponton LE, editors. Handbook of adolescent health risk behavior. Berlin: Springer Science & Business Media; 1996. p. 35–51.

62. Resch F, Westhoff K. Das biopsychosoziale Modell in der Praxis: Eine kritische Reflexion. Resonanzen. 2013;1:32–46.

63. Resch F, Westhoff K. Wie weit trägt das biopsychosoziale Modell des Menschen in der Psychotherapie? Psychotherapie Forum. 2006;14:186–92. https://doi.org/10.1007/s00729-006-0167-9.
64. Resch F, Westhoff K. Neuromythologien und das Dilemma des biopsychosozialen Modells. Zeitschrift für Individualpsychologie. 2008a;33:140–7.
65. Fuchs T. Verteidigung des Menschen: Grundfragen einer verkörperten Anthropologie. Frankfurt a.M: Suhrkamp Verlag; 2020.
66. Sullivan CJ, Childs KK, O'Connell D. Adolescent risk behavior subgroups: an empirical assessment. J Youth Adolesc. 2010;39:541–62. https://doi.org/10.1007/s10964-009-9445-5.
67. Wasserman D, Carli V, Wasserman C, et al. Saving and empowering young lives in Europe (SEYLE): a randomized controlled trial. BMC Public Health. 2010;10:192. https://doi.org/10.1186/1471-2458-10-192.
68. Wasserman D, Hoven CW, Wasserman C, et al. School-based suicide prevention programmes: the SEYLE cluster-randomised, controlled trial. Lancet. 2015;385:1536–44. https://doi.org/10.1016/S0140-6736(14)61213-7.
69. Carli V, Hoven CW, Wasserman C, et al. A newly identified group of adolescents at "invisible" risk for psychopathology and suicidal behavior: findings from the SEYLE study. World Psychiatry. 2014;13:78–86. https://doi.org/10.1002/wps.20088.
70. Kaess M, Parzer P, Brunner R, et al. Pathological internet use is on the rise among European adolescents. J Adolesc Health. 2016;59:236–9. https://doi.org/10.1016/j.jadohealth.2016.04.009.
71. Gentile DA, Bailey K, Bavelier D, et al. Internet gaming disorder in children and adolescents. Pediatrics. 2017;140:S81–5. https://doi.org/10.1542/peds.2016-1758H.
72. Mihara S, Higuchi S. Cross-sectional and longitudinal epidemiological studies of Internet gaming disorder: a systematic review of the literature. Psychiatry Clin Neurosci. 2017;71:425–44. https://doi.org/10.1111/pcn.12532.
73. Young K, Pistner M, O'Mara J, Buchanan J. Cyber disorders: the mental health concern for the new millennium. Cyberpsychol Behav. 1999;2:475–9. https://doi.org/10.1089/cpb.1999.2.475.
74. American Psychiatric Association. Diagnostisches und Statistisches Manual Psychischer Störungen—DSM-5. Göttingen: Hogrefe; 2015.
75. Touitou Y, Touitou D, Reinberg A. Disruption of adolescents' circadian clock: the vicious circle of media use, exposure to light at night, sleep loss and risk behaviors. J Physiol Paris. 2016;110:467–79. https://doi.org/10.1016/j.jphysparis.2017.05.001.
76. Durkee T, Kaess M, Carli V, et al. Prevalence of pathological internet use among adolescents in Europe: demographic and social factors. Addiction. 2012;107:2210–22. https://doi.org/10.1111/j.1360-0443.2012.03946.x.
77. Strittmatter E, Kaess M, Parzer P, et al. Pathological Internet use among adolescents: comparing gamers and non-gamers. Psychiatry Res. 2015;228:128–35. https://doi.org/10.1016/j.psychres.2015.04.029.
78. von Salisch M. Beschäftigung mit gewalthaltigen Computerspielen und offen aggressives Verhalten bei Kindern und Jugendlichen: Ein Literaturüberblick zur Wirkrichtung. Prax Kinderpsychol Kinderpsychiatr. 2020;69:109–25. https://doi.org/10.13109/prkk.2020.69.2.109.
79. Prescott AT, Sargent JD, Hull JG. Metaanalysis of the relationship between violent video game play and physical aggression over time. Proc Natl Acad Sci U S A. 2018;115:9882–8. https://doi.org/10.1073/pnas.1611617114.
80. Štulhofer A, Tafro A, Kohut T. The dynamics of adolescents' pornography use and psychological well-being: a six-wave latent growth and latent class modeling approach. Eur Child Adolesc Psychiatry. 2019;28:1567–79. https://doi.org/10.1007/s00787-019-01318-4.
81. Sohn S, Rees P, Wildridge B, et al. Prevalence of problematic smartphone usage and associated mental health outcomes amongst children and young people: a systematic review, meta-analysis and GRADE of the evidence. BMC Psychiatry. 2019;19:356. https://doi.org/10.1186/s12888-019-2350-x.
82. Finkelhor D, Browne A. The traumatic impact of child sexual abuse: a conceptualization. Am J Orthopsychiatry. 1985;55:530–41. https://doi.org/10.1111/j.1939-0025.1985.tb02703.x.

83. Jones DJ, Lewis T, Litrownik A, et al. Linking childhood sexual abuse and early adolescent risk behavior: the intervening role of internalizing and externalizing problems. J Abnorm Child Psychol. 2013;41:139–50. https://doi.org/10.1007/s10802-012-9656-1.

84. Jordan CJ, Andersen SL. Sensitive periods of substance abuse: early risk for the transition to dependence. Dev Cogn Neurosci. 2017;25:29–44. https://doi.org/10.1016/j.dcn.2016.10.004.

85. Welch KA, Carson A, Lawrie SM. Brain structure in adolescents and young adults with alcohol problems: systematic review of imaging studies. Alcohol Alcohol. 2013;48:433–44. https://doi.org/10.1093/alcalc/agt037.

86. Banzer R, Haring C, Buchheim A, et al. Factors associated with different smoking status in European adolescents: results of the SEYLE study. Eur Child Adolesc Psychiatry. 2017;26:1319–29. https://doi.org/10.1007/s00787-017-0980-4.

87. Ambrose BK, Day HR, Rostron B, et al. Flavored tobacco product use among US youth aged 12–17 years, 2013–2014. JAMA. 2015;314:1871–3. https://doi.org/10.1001/jama.2015.13802.

88. Romer D, Moreno M. Digital media and risks for adolescent substance abuse and problematic gambling. Pediatrics. 2017;140:S102–6. https://doi.org/10.1542/peds.2016-1758L.

89. Jawad M, Charide R, Waziry R, et al. The prevalence and trends of waterpipe tobacco smoking: a systematic review. PLoS One. 2018;13:e0192191. https://doi.org/10.1371/journal.pone.0192191.

90. Kotz D, Kastaun S. E-Zigaretten und Tabakerhitzer: repräsentative Daten zu Konsumverhalten und assoziierten Faktoren in der deutschen Bevölkerung (die DEBRA-Studie). Bundesgesundheitsbl. 2018;61:1407–14. https://doi.org/10.1007/s00103-018-2827-7.

91. Ghinea D, Parzer P, Resch F, et al. Zusammenhänge von Drogenkonsum und der Borderline-Persönlichkeitsstörung sowie Depressivität in einer klinischen Stichprobe an Jugendlichen. Prax Kinderpsychol Kinderpsychiatr. 2020b;69:126–40. https://doi.org/10.13109/prkk.2020.69.2.126.

92. Resch F. Der Körper als Instrument zur Bewältigung seelischer Krisen: Selbstverletzendes Verhalten bei Jugendlichen. Dtsch Arztbl. 2001;98:2266–71.

93. Plener PL, Libal G, Keller F, et al. An international comparison of adolescent non-suicidal self-injury (NSSI) and suicide attempts: Germany and the USA. Psychol Med. 2009;39:1549–58. https://doi.org/10.1017/S0033291708005114.

94. Brunner R, Parzer P, Haffner J, et al. Prevalence and psychological correlates of occasional and repetitive deliberate self-harm in adolescents. Arch Pediatr Adolesc Med. 2007;161:641–9. https://doi.org/10.1001/archpedi.161.7.641.

95. Resch F. Selbstverletzung als Selbstfürsorge: Zur Psychodynamik selbstschädigenden Verhaltens bei Jugendlichen. 1st ed. Göttingen: Vandenhoeck & Ruprecht; 2017a.

96. Resch F, Kaess M, Plener PL, Fegert JM. Suizidales Verhalten. In: Fegert JM, Eggers C, Resch F, editors. Psychiatrie und Psychotherapie des Kindes- und Jugendalters. 2nd ed. Heidelberg: Springer; 2012. p. 959–70.

97. Plener P, Brunner R, Resch F, et al. Selbstverletzendes Verhalten im Jugendalter. Z Kinder Jugendpsychiatr Psychother. 2010;38:77–89. https://doi.org/10.1024/1422-4917.a000015.

98. Guan K, Fox KR, Prinstein MJ. Nonsuicidal self-injury as a time-invariant predictor of adolescent suicide ideation and attempts in a diverse community sample. J Consult Clin Psychol. 2012;80:842–9. https://doi.org/10.1037/a0029429.

99. Hartley CM, Pettit JW, Castellanos D. Reactive aggression and suicide-related behaviors in children and adolescents: a review and preliminary meta-analysis. Suicide Life Threat Behav. 2018;48:38–51. https://doi.org/10.1111/sltb.12325.

100. Zetterqvist M, Lundh L-G, Svedin CG. A cross-sectional study of adolescent non-suicidal self-injury: support for a specific distress-function relationship. Child Adolesc Psychiatry Ment Health. 2014;8:23. https://doi.org/10.1186/1753-2000-8-23.

101. Kaess M, Parzer P, Mattern M, et al. Adverse childhood experiences and their impact on frequency, severity, and the individual function of nonsuicidal self-injury in youth. Psychiatry Res. 2013;206:265–72. https://doi.org/10.1016/j.psychres.2012.10.012.

102. Ghinea D, Koenig J, Parzer P, et al. Longitudinal development of risk-taking and self-injurious behavior in association with late adolescent borderline personality disorder symptoms. Psychiatry Res. 2019;273:127–33. https://doi.org/10.1016/j.psychres.2019.01.010.

103. Ghinea D, Edinger A, Parzer P, et al. Non-suicidal self-injury disorder as a stand-alone diagnosis in a consecutive help-seeking sample of adolescents. J Affect Disord. 2020a;274:1122–5. https://doi.org/10.1016/j.jad.2020.06.009.

104. Cohrdes C, Göbel K, Schlack R, Hölling H. Essstörungssymptome bei Kindern und Jugendlichen: Häufigkeiten und Risikofaktoren. Bundesgesundheitsbl. 2019;62:1195–204. https://doi.org/10.1007/s00103-019-03005-w.

105. Schuck K, Munsch S, Schneider S. Body image perceptions and symptoms of disturbed eating behavior among children and adolescents in Germany. Child Adolesc Psychiatry Ment Health. 2018;12:10. https://doi.org/10.1186/s13034-018-0216-5.

106. Weissman RS. The role of sociocultural factors in the etiology of eating disorders. Psychiatr Clin North Am. 2019;42:121–44. https://doi.org/10.1016/j.psc.2018.10.009.

107. Boucher K, Côté M, Gagnon-Girouard M-P, et al. Eating pathology among patients with Anorexia Nervosa and Bulimia Nervosa: the role of narcissism and self-esteem. J Nerv Ment Dis. 2018;206:776–82. https://doi.org/10.1097/NMD.0000000000000890.

108. Tremblay RE. The development of aggressive behaviour during childhood: what have we learned in the past century? Int J Behav Dev. 2000;24:129–41. https://doi.org/10.1080/016502500383232.

109. Cleverley K, Szatmari P, Vaillancourt T, et al. Developmental trajectories of physical and indirect aggression from late childhood to adolescence: sex differences and outcomes in emerging adulthood. J Am Acad Child Adolesc Psychiatry. 2012;51:1037–51. https://doi.org/10.1016/j.jaac.2012.07.010.

110. Loeber R, Burke JD, Pardini DA. Development and etiology of disruptive and delinquent behavior. Annu Rev Clin Psychol. 2009;5:291–310. https://doi.org/10.1146/annurev.clinpsy.032408.153631.

111. Moffitt TE. Adolescence-limited and life-course-persistent antisocial behavior: a developmental taxonomy. Psychol Rev. 1993;100:674–701.

112. Assink M, van der Put CE, Hoeve M, et al. Risk factors for persistent delinquent behavior among juveniles: a meta-analytic review. Clin Psychol Rev. 2015;42:47–61. https://doi.org/10.1016/j.cpr.2015.08.002.

113. Fairchild G, van Goozen SHM, Calder AJ, Goodyer IM. Research review: evaluating and reformulating the developmental taxonomic theory of antisocial behaviour. J Child Psychol Psychiatry. 2013;54:924–40. https://doi.org/10.1111/jcpp.12102.

114. Carlisi CO, Moffitt TE, Knodt AR, et al. Associations between life-course-persistent antisocial behaviour and brain structure in a population-representative longitudinal birth cohort. Lancet Psychiatry. 2020;7:245–53. https://doi.org/10.1016/S2215-0366(20)30002-X.

115. Heerde JA, Hemphill SA. Sexual risk behaviors, sexual offenses, and sexual victimization among homeless youth: a systematic review of associations with substance use. Trauma Violence Abuse. 2016;17:468–89. https://doi.org/10.1177/1524838015584371.

116. Samkange-Zeeb FN, Spallek L, Zeeb H. Awareness and knowledge of sexually transmitted diseases (STDs) among school-going adolescents in Europe: a systematic review of published literature. BMC Public Health. 2011;11:727. https://doi.org/10.1186/1471-2458-11-727.

117. McClellan K, Temples H, Miller L. The latest in teen pregnancy prevention: long-acting reversible contraception. J Pediatr Health Care. 2018;32:e91–7. https://doi.org/10.1016/j.pedhc.2018.02.009.

118. McCracken KA, Loveless M. Teen pregnancy: an update. Curr Opin Obstet Gynecol. 2014;26:355–9. https://doi.org/10.1097/GCO.0000000000000102.

119. Reck C, Backenstrass M, Möhler E, et al. Mutter-Kind-Interaktion und postpartale Depression: Theorie und Empirie im Überblick. Psychother Psych Med. 2001;6:171–86.

120. Huang CY, Costeines J, Ayala C, Kaufman JS. Parenting stress, social support, and depression for ethnic minority adolescent mothers: impact on child development. J Child Fam Stud. 2014;23:255–62. https://doi.org/10.1007/s10826-013-9807-1.
121. Lindberg L, Santelli J, Desai S. Understanding the decline in adolescent fertility in the United States, 2007–2012. J Adolesc Health. 2016;59:577–83. https://doi.org/10.1016/j.jadohealth.2016.06.024.
122. Craig W, Harel-Fisch Y, Fogel-Grinvald H, et al. A cross-national profile of bullying and victimization among adolescents in 40 countries. Int J Public Health. 2009;54(Suppl 2):216–24. https://doi.org/10.1007/s00038-009-5413-9.
123. Jantzer V, Haffner J, Parzer P, Resch F. Opfer von Bullying in der Schule: Depressivität, Suizidalität und selbstverletzendes Verhalten bei deutschen Jugendlichen. Kindh Entwickl. 2012;21:40–6. https://doi.org/10.1026/0942-5403/a000068.
124. Jantzer V, Schlander M, Haffner J, et al. The cost incurred by victims of bullying from a societal perspective: estimates based on a German online survey of adolescents. Eur Child Adolesc Psychiatry. 2019;28:585–94. https://doi.org/10.1007/s00787-018-1224-y.
125. Allen CW, Diamond-Myrsten S, Rollins LK. School absenteeism in children and adolescents. Am Fam Physician. 2018;98:738–44.
126. Kearney CA. School absenteeism and school refusal behavior in youth: a contemporary review. Clin Psychol Rev. 2008;28:451–71. https://doi.org/10.1016/j.cpr.2007.07.012.
127. Gubbels J, van der Put CE, Assink M. Risk factors for school absenteeism and dropout: a meta-analytic review. J Youth Adolesc. 2019;48:1637–67. https://doi.org/10.1007/s10964-019-01072-5.
128. Lenzen C, Brunner R, Resch F. Schulabsentismus: Entwicklungen und fortbestehende Herausforderungen. Z Kinder Jugendpsychiatr Psychother. 2016;44:101–11. https://doi.org/10.1024/1422-4917/a000405.
129. Resch F. Entwicklungspsychopathologie des Kindes- und Jugendalters: ein Lehrbuch. Weinheim: Beltz; 1999a.
130. Resch F. Entwicklungspsychopathologie. In: Fegert J, Resch F, Döpfner M, et al., editors. Psychiatrie und Psychotherapie des Kindes- und Jugendalterns. Heidelberg: Springer; 2021a.
131. Cicchetti D, Cohen DJ. Developmental psychopathology. New York: Wiley; 1995.
132. Petermann F, Resch F. Entwicklungspsychopathologie. In: Petermann F, editor. Lehrbuch der Klinischen Kinderpsychologie. 7th ed. Göttingen: Hogrefe; 2013. p. 57–76.
133. Pollak SD. Developmental psychopathology: recent advances and future challenges. World Psychiatry. 2015;14:262–9. https://doi.org/10.1002/wps.20237.
134. Resch F. Beitrag der klinischen Entwicklungspsychologie zu einem neuen Verständnis von Normalität und Pathologie. In: Oerter R, von Hagen C, Röper G, Noam G, editors. Klinische Entwicklungspsychologie: Ein Lehrbuch. Weinheim: Beltz; 1999b. p. 606–22.
135. Rutter M, Sroufe LA. Developmental psychopathology: concepts and challenges. Dev Psychopathol. 2000;12:265–96.
136. Wille N, Bettge S, Ravens-Sieberer U, BELLA Study Group. Risk and protective factors for children's and adolescents' mental health: results of the BELLA study. Eur Child Adolesc Psychiatry. 2008;17(Suppl 1):133–47. https://doi.org/10.1007/s00787-008-1015-y.
137. Antonovsky A. Unraveling the mystery of health. 1st ed. San Francisco: Jossey-Bass; 1987.
138. Werner EE, Smith RS. Journeys from childhood to midlife: risk, resilience, and recovery. Ithaca: Cornell University Press; 2001.
139. Feldman R. What is resilience: an affiliative neuroscience approach. World Psychiatry. 2020;19:132–50. https://doi.org/10.1002/wps.20729.
140. Damasio AR. Ich fühle, also bin ich: die Entschlüsselung des Bewusstseins. München: List Taschenbuch; 2013.
141. Resch F, Freyberger H. Struktur und Identität. In: Fegert JM, Streeck-Fischer A, Freyberger H, editors. Adoleszenzpsychiatrie. Psychiatrie und Psychotherapie der Adoleszenz und des jungen Erwachsenenalters. Stuttgart: Schattauer; 2009. p. 105–11.

142. Resch F, Koch E. Bedeutung der Strukturachse für Therapieplanung und Behandlung. Kinderanalyse. 2012;20:4–20.
143. Stern DN. The interpersonal world of the infant. New York: Basic Books; 1985.
144. Fonagy P, Gergely G, Jurist EL, Target M. Affektregulierung, Mentalisierung und die Entwicklung des Selbst. Stuttgart: Klett-Cotta; 2006.
145. Cicchetti D. Annual research review: resilient functioning in maltreated children—past, present, and future perspectives. J Child Psychol Psychiatry. 2013;54:402–22. https://doi.org/10.1111/j.1469-7610.2012.02608.x.
146. Campos JJ, Stenberg C. Perception, appraisal, and emotion: the onset of social referencing. In: Lamb ME, Sherrod LR, editors. Infant social cognition: empirical and theoretical considerations. Hillsdale: Lawrence Erlbaum Associates; 1981. p. 273–314.
147. Resch F. Entwicklungspsychopathologie der frühen Kindheit im interdisziplinären Spannungsfeld. In: Papoušek M, Schieche M, Wurmser H, editors. Regulationsstörungen der frühen Kindheit: frühe Risiken und Hilfen im Entwicklungskontext der Eltern-Kind-Beziehungen. Bern: Huber; 2004. p. 31–47.
148. Hyde LW. Developmental psychopathology in an era of molecular genetics and neuroimaging: a developmental neurogenetics approach. Dev Psychopathol. 2015;27:587–613. https://doi.org/10.1017/S0954579415000188.
149. Siegel DJ. The developing mind: how relationships and the brain interact to shape who we are. New York: Guilford Press; 1999.
150. Ciompi L. Affektlogik: über die Struktur der Psyche und ihre Entwicklung: ein Beitrag zur Schizophrenieforschung. Stuttgart: Klett-Cotta; 1982.
151. Fegert JM, Resch F. Risiko, Vulnerabilität, Resilienz und Prävention. In: Fegert JM, Eggers C, Resch F, editors. Psychiatrie und Psychotherapie des Kindes-und Jugendalters. 2nd ed. Berlin: Springer; 2012. p. 131–42.
152. Resch F, Fegert JM. Ätilogische Modelle. In: Fegert JM, Eggers C, Resch F, editors. Psychiatrie und Psychotherapie des Kindes- und Jugendalters. 2nd ed. Berlin: Springer; 2012. p. 115–30.
153. Perry BD, Pollard RA, Blakley TL, et al. Kindheitstrauma, Neurobiologie der Anpassung und "gebrauchsabhängige" Entwicklung des Gehirns: Wie "Zustände" zu "Eigenschaften" werden. Analytische Kinder- und Jugendlichen-Psychotherapie. 1998;29:277–307.
154. Sachsse U. Hinterlassen seelische Schädigungen in der Kindheit neurobiologische Spuren im erwachsenen Gehirn? Prax Kinderpsychol Kinderpsychiatr. 2013;62:778–92.
155. Resch F. Kinder- und Jugendmedizin. In: Köhle K, Herzog W, Joraschky P, et al., editors. Uexküll, psychosomatische Medizin theoretische Modelle und klinische Praxis. 8th ed. München: Elsevier; 2017b. p. 1099–111.
156. Siever LJ. Neurobiology of aggression and violence. Am J Psychiatry. 2008;165:429–42. https://doi.org/10.1176/appi.ajp.2008.07111774.
157. Brumariu LE. Parent-child attachment and emotion regulation. New Dir Child Adolesc Dev. 2015;2015:31–45. https://doi.org/10.1002/cad.20098.
158. Shonkoff JP, Garner AS, Committee on Psychosocial Aspects of Child and Family Health, et al. The lifelong effects of early childhood adversity and toxic stress. Pediatrics. 2012;129:e232–46. https://doi.org/10.1542/peds.2011-2663.
159. Terr LC. Childhood traumas: an outline and overview. Am J Psychiatry. 1991;148:10–20.
160. Fuchs A, Führer D, Bierbaum A-L, et al. Transgenerationale Einflussfaktoren kindlicher Inhibitionskontrolle: Mütterliche Traumaerfahrung, Depression und Impulsivität. Prax Kinderpsychol Kinderpsychiatr. 2016;65:423–40. https://doi.org/10.13109/prkk.2016.65.6.423.
161. Kluczniok D, Boedeker K, Fuchs A, et al. Emotional availability in mother-child interaction: the effects of maternal depression in remission and additional history of childhood abuse. Depress Anxiety. 2016;33:648–57. https://doi.org/10.1002/da.22462.
162. Moehler E, Biringen Z, Poustka L. Emotional availability in a sample of mothers with a history of abuse. Am J Orthopsychiatry. 2007;77:624–8. https://doi.org/10.1037/0002-9432.77.4.624.

163. Zeanah CH, Scheeringa M, Boris NW, et al. Reactive attachment disorder in maltreated toddlers. Child Abuse Negl. 2004;28:877–88. https://doi.org/10.1016/j.chiabu.2004.01.010.
164. Möhler E, Matheis V, Poustka L, et al. Mothers with a history of abuse tend to show more impulsiveness. Child Abuse Negl. 2009;33:123–6. https://doi.org/10.1016/j.chiabu.2008.06.002.
165. Felitti VJ. Long-term medical consequences of incest, rape, and molestation. South Med J. 1991;84:328–31. https://doi.org/10.1097/00007611-199103000-00008.
166. Huang H, Yan P, Shan Z, et al. Adverse childhood experiences and risk of type 2 diabetes: a systematic review and meta-analysis. Metab Clin Exp. 2015;64:1408–18. https://doi.org/10.1016/j.metabol.2015.08.019.
167. Norman RE, Byambaa M, De R, et al. The long-term health consequences of child physical abuse, emotional abuse, and neglect: a systematic review and meta-analysis. PLoS Med. 2012;9:e1001349. https://doi.org/10.1371/journal.pmed.1001349.
168. Felitti VJ, Anda RF, Nordenberg D, et al. Relationship of childhood abuse and household dysfunction to many of the leading causes of death in adults. The Adverse Childhood Experiences (ACE) Study. Am J Prev Med. 1998;14:245–58. https://doi.org/10.1016/s0749-3797(98)00017-8.
169. Lazarus RS. Progress on a cognitive-motivational-relational theory of emotion. Am Psychol. 1991;46:819–34. https://doi.org/10.1037//0003-066x.46.8.819.
170. Gross JJ. Emotion regulation: affective, cognitive, and social consequences. Psychophysiology. 2002;39:281–91. https://doi.org/10.1017/s0048577201393198.
171. Frijda NH. The emotions. Cambridge: Cambridge University Press; 1986.
172. LeDoux JE. Emotion: clues from the brain. Annu Rev Psychol. 1995;46:209–35. https://doi.org/10.1146/annurev.ps.46.020195.001233.
173. John OP, Gross JJ. Healthy and unhealthy emotion regulation: personality processes, individual differences, and life span development. J Pers. 2004;72:1301–33. https://doi.org/10.1111/j.1467-6494.2004.00298.x.
174. Kullik A, Petermann F. Emotionsregulation im Kindesalter. Göttingen: Hogrefe Verlag; 2012.
175. Kerr KL, Ratliff EL, Cosgrove KT, et al. Parental influences on neural mechanisms underlying emotion regulation. Trends Neurosci Educ. 2019;16:100118. https://doi.org/10.1016/j.tine.2019.100118.
176. Young KS, Sandman CF, Craske MG. Positive and negative emotion regulation in adolescence: links to anxiety and depression. Brain Sci. 2019;9:76. https://doi.org/10.3390/brainsci9040076.
177. Moltrecht B, Deighton J, Patalay P, Edbrooke-Childs J. Effectiveness of current psychological interventions to improve emotion regulation in youth: a meta-analysis. Eur Child Adolesc Psychiatry. 2020; https://doi.org/10.1007/s00787-020-01498-4.
178. Oerter R, Montada L, editors. Entwicklungspsychologie: ein Lehrbuch. 3rd ed. Weinheim: Beltz; 1995.
179. Bischof N. Struktur und Bedeutung: eine Einführung in die Systemtheorie. Bern: Huber; 2013.
180. Powers WT. Behavior: the control of perception. Chicago: Aldine; 1973a.
181. Schleiffer R. Verhaltensstörungen: Sinn und Funktion. Heidelberg: Carl Auer Verlag; 2013.
182. Freud S. Wege der psychoanalytischen Therapie. In: Gesammelte Werke XII. Frankfurt: Fischer; 1919. p. 183–94.
183. Skinner BF. Contingencies of reinforcement: a theoretical analysis. New York: Appleton-Century-Crofts; 1969.
184. Herpertz-Dahlmann B, Resch F, Schulte-Markwort M, Warnke A. Entwicklungspsychiatrie. In: Herpertz-Dahlmann B, Resch F, Schulte-Markwort M, Warnke A, editors. Entwicklungspsychiatrie: Biopsychologische Grundlagen und die Entwicklung psychischer Störungen. 2nd ed. Stuttgart: Schattauer; 2008. p. 303–51.
185. Caspi A, McClay J, Moffitt TE, et al. Role of genotype in the cycle of violence in maltreated children. Science. 2002;297:851–4. https://doi.org/10.1126/science.1072290.
186. Caspi A, Moffitt TE. Gene-environment interactions in psychiatry: joining forces with neuroscience. Nat Rev Neurosci. 2006;7:583–90. https://doi.org/10.1038/nrn1925.

187. Feder A, Nestler EJ, Charney DS. Psychobiology and molecular genetics of resilience. Nat Rev Neurosci. 2009;10:446–57. https://doi.org/10.1038/nrn2649.
188. Kinnally EL, Huang Y, Haverly R, et al. Parental care moderates the influence of MAOA-uVNTR genotype and childhood stressors on trait impulsivity and aggression in adult women. Psychiatr Genet. 2009;19:126–33. https://doi.org/10.1097/YPG.0b013e32832a50a7.
189. Reichl C, Kaess M, Resch F, Brunner R. Die Rolle des Genotyps bei der generationsübergreifenden Übertragung belastender Kindheitserlebnisse. Z Kinder Jugendpsychiatr Psychother. 2014;42:349–59. https://doi.org/10.1024/1422-4917/a000310.
190. Kieling C, Hutz MH, Genro JP, et al. Gene-environment interaction in externalizing problems among adolescents: evidence from the Pelotas 1993 Birth Cohort Study. J Child Psychol Psychiatry. 2013;54:298–304. https://doi.org/10.1111/jcpp.12022.
191. Sturma D. Philosophie und Neurowissenschaften. Frankfurt: Suhrkamp; 2006.
192. Fuchs T. Das Gehirn - ein Beziehungsorgan: Eine phänomenologisch-ökologische Konzeption. Stuttgart: Kohlhammer; 2017.
193. Wittgenstein L. Philosophische Untersuchungen. Frankfurt: Suhrkamp; 1978.
194. Resch F, Parzer P. Gibt es psychopathologische Modelle zur Erklärung der Wirkungen von Psychotherapie und Psychopharmakotherapie? In: Küchenhoff J, editor. Psychopharmakologie und Psychoanalyse. Grundlagen, Klinik, Forschung. Stuttgart: Kohlhammer; 2016. p. 72–90.
195. Herpertz S, Caspar F, Mundt C, editors. Störungsorientierte Psychotherapie. München: Urban & Fischer; 2008.
196. Bastine R. Komorbidität: Ein Anachronismus und eine Herausforderung für die Psychotherapie. In: Fiedler P, editor. Die Zukunft der Psychotherapie. Heidelberg: Springer; 2012. p. 13–26.
197. Resch F. Die Perspektive der Kindheit und Jugend. In: Fiedler P, editor. Die Zukunft der Psychotherapie. Heidelberg: Springer; 2012. p. 93–116.
198. Resch F. Struktur und Strukturveränderungen im Kindes- und Jugendalter. In: Rudolf G, Grande T, Henningsen P, editors. Die Struktur der Persönlichkeit. Stuttgart: Vom theoretischen Verständnis zur psychotherapeutischen Anwendung des psychodynamischen Strukturkonzepts. Schattauer; 2002. p. 116–31.
199. Resch F. Developing mind: Intersubjektivität und die Entwicklung der psychischen Struktur. In: Resch F, Schulte-Markwort M, editors. Kindheit im digitalen Zeitalter. Weinheim: Beltz; 2009. p. 2–22.
200. Frank M. Selbstbewusstsein und Selbsterkenntnis: Essays zur analytischen Philosophie der Subjektivität. Stuttgart: P. Reclam; 1991.
201. Damon W, Hart D. The development of self-understanding from infancy through adolescence. Child Dev. 1982;53:841–64. https://doi.org/10.2307/1129122.
202. Resch F. Tiefenpsychologische Diagnostik. In: Fegert J, Resch F, Döpfner M, et al., editors. Psychiatrie und Psychotherapie des Kindes- und Jugendalterns. Heidelberg: Springer; 2021b.
203. Resch F, Möhler E. Wie entwickelt sich die kindliche Persönlichkeit? Beiträge zur Diskussion um Vererbung und Umwelt. In: Bartram CR, Wink M, editors. Vererbung und Milieu. Heidelberg: Springer; 2001. p. 95–151.
204. Powers WT. Living control systems: selected papers of William T. Powers. Gravel Switch, KY: The Control Systems Group; 1989.
205. Squire LR. The neuropsychology of human memory. Annu Rev Neurosci. 1982;5:241–73. https://doi.org/10.1146/annurev.ne.05.030182.001325.
206. Markowitsch HJ. Das Gedächtnis: Entwicklung, Funktionen, Störungen. München: Beck; 2009.
207. Fonagy P, Target M, Allison L. Gedächtnis und therapeutische Wirkung. Psyche. 2003;57:841–56.
208. Dornes M. Über Mentalisierung, Affektregulierung und die Entwicklung des Selbst. Forum Psychoanal. 2004;20:175–99.
209. Fuchs T, De Jaegher H. Non-representational intersubjectivity. Vortrag präsentiert bei der DISCOS International Conference; 2008.

210. Fuchs T. Ecology of the brain: the phenomenology and biology of the embodied mind. Oxford: Oxford University Press; 2018.
211. Fonagy P, Target M. Mit der Realität spielen. Zur Doppelgesichtigkeit psychischer Realität von Borderline-Patienten. Psyche. 2001;55:961–95.
212. Kernberg OF. Schwere Persönlichkeitsstörungen. Stuttgart: Klett-Cotta; 1988.
213. O'Brien WH, Carhart V. Functional analysis in behavioral medicine. Eur J Psychol Assess. 2011;27:4–16. https://doi.org/10.1027/1015-5759/a000052.
214. Hayes SC, Strosahl KD, Wilson KG. Acceptance and commitment therapy: an experiential approach to behavior change. New York: Guilford Press; 1999.
215. Linehan MM, Comtois KA, Murray AM, et al. Two-year randomized controlled trial and follow-up of dialectical behavior therapy vs therapy by experts for suicidal behaviors and borderline personality disorder. Arch Gen Psychiatry. 2006;63:757–66. https://doi.org/10.1001/archpsyc.63.7.757.
216. Kohlenberg R, Kanter J, Bolling M, et al. Functional analytic psychotherapy, cognitive therapy, and acceptance. In: Hayes SC, Follette VM, Linehan MM, editors. Mindfulness and acceptance: expanding the cognitive-behavioral tradition. New York: Guilford Press; 2011. p. 96–119.
217. Segal ZV, Williams MG, Teasdale JD. Mindfulness-based cognitive therapy for depression. New York: Guilford Press; 2013.
218. Hayes SC. Acceptance and commitment therapy, relational frame theory, and the third wave of behavioral and cognitive therapies. Behav Ther. 2004;35:639–65. https://doi.org/10.1016/S0005-7894(04)80013-3.
219. Sannwald R, Resch F, Schulte-Markwort M. Psychotherapeutische Fertigkeiten. Göttingen: Vandenhoeck & Ruprecht; 2013.
220. von Sydow K. Systemische Psychotherapie (mit Familien, Paaren und Einzelnen). In: Reimer C, Eckert J, Hautzinger M, Wilke E, editors. Psychotherapie: Ein Lehrbuch für Ärzte und Psychologen. 3rd ed. Heidelberg: Springer; 2007. p. 289–316.
221. Grawe K. Psychologische Therapie. Göttingen: Hogrefe; 2000.
222. Marken RS. You say you had a revolution: methodological foundations of closed-loop psychology. Rev Gen Psychol. 2009;13:137–45. https://doi.org/10.1037/a0015106.
223. Ashby RW. Mechanisms of intelligence. Seaside, CA: Intersystems Publications; 1981.
224. von Bertalanffy L. General system theory; foundations, development, applications. New York: G. Braziller; 1969.
225. Wiener N. Cybernetics; or, control and communication in the animal and the machine. New York: MIT Press; 1961.
226. Powers WT. Feedback: beyond behaviorism: stimulus-response laws are wholly predictable within a control-system model of behavioral organization. Science. 1973b;179:351–6. https://doi.org/10.1126/science.179.4071.351.
227. Baum WM, Reese HW, Powers WT. Behaviorism and feedback control. Science. 1973;181:1114–20.
228. Carver CS, Scheier M. On the self-regulation of behavior. Cambridge: Cambridge University Press; 1998.
229. Marken RS, Powers WT. Random-walk chemotaxis: trial and error as a control process. Behav Neurosci. 1989;103:1348–55. https://doi.org/10.1037//0735-7044.103.6.1348.
230. Mansell W. Understanding control and utilizing control theory in the science and practice of CBT. Cogn Behav Therapist. 2009;2:115–7. https://doi.org/10.1017/S1754470X09990146.
231. Carey TA, Kelly RE, Mansell W, Tai SJ. What's therapeutic about the therapeutic relationship? A hypothesis for practice informed by Perceptual Control Theory. Cogn Behav Therapist. 2012;5:47–59. https://doi.org/10.1017/S1754470X12000037.
232. Müller-Fries E, Hellhammer D, Lehnert H, Kirschbaum C. Psychoneuroendokrinologie. In: Köhle K, Herzog W, Joraschky P, et al., editors. Uexküll: Psychosomatische Medizin: theoretische Modelle und klinische Praxis. München: Elsevier; 2017. p. 57–63.
233. Dyslin CW. Perceptual control theory: a model of volitional behavior in accord with the ideas of Alfred Adler. J Individ Psychol. 1998;54:24–40.

234. Adler A. Praxis und Theorie der Individualpsychologie. Frankfurt: Fischer; 1978.
235. Young JE, Klosko JS, Weishaar ME. Schematherapie. Ein praxisorientiertes Handbuch. 2nd ed. Paderborn: Junfermann Verlag; 2008.
236. Rudolf G. Strukturbezogene Psychotherapie: Leitfaden zur psychodynamischen Therapie struktureller Störungen. 3rd ed. Stuttgart: Schattauer; 2012.
237. Ruge E. Metropol. Frankfurt a.M: Büchergilde Gutenberg; 2019.
238. Schlack HG, Brockmann K. Einfluss sozialer Faktoren auf Gesundheit und Entwicklung von Kindern. In: Hoffmann GF, Lentze MJ, Spranger J, Zepp F, editors. Pädiatrie—Grundlagen und Praxis. 4th ed. Berlin: Springer; 2014. p. 152–5.
239. Ravens-Sieberer U, Otto C, Kriston L, et al. The longitudinal BELLA study: design, methods and first results on the course of mental health problems. Eur Child Adolesc Psychiatry. 2015;24:651–63. https://doi.org/10.1007/s00787-014-0638-4.
240. Barkmann C, Schulte-Markwort M. Prävalenz psychischer Auffälligkeit bei Kindern und Jugendlichen in Deutschland—ein systematischer Literaturüberblick. Psychiatr Prax. 2004;31:278–87. https://doi.org/10.1055/s-2003-814855.
241. Atladottir HO, Gyllenberg D, Langridge A, et al. The increasing prevalence of reported diagnoses of childhood psychiatric disorders: a descriptive multinational comparison. Eur Child Adolesc Psychiatry. 2015;24:173–83. https://doi.org/10.1007/s00787-014-0553-8.
242. Hawton K, Saunders KEA, O'Connor RC. Self-harm and suicide in adolescents. Lancet. 2012;379:2373–82. https://doi.org/10.1016/S0140-6736(12)60322-5.
243. Costello EJ. Commentary: "Diseases of the world": from epidemiology to etiology of child and adolescent psychopathology—a commentary on Polanczyk et al. (2015). J Child Psychol Psychiatry. 2015;56:366–9. https://doi.org/10.1111/jcpp.12402.
244. Carpentier MY, Mullins LL, Elkin TD, Wolfe-Christensen C. Prevalence of multiple health-related behaviors in adolescents with cancer. J Pediatr Hematol Oncol. 2008;30:902–7. https://doi.org/10.1097/MPH.0b013e318186533f.
245. Van Lieshout RJ, Boyle MH, Saigal S, et al. Mental health of extremely low birth weight survivors in their 30s. Pediatrics. 2015;135:452–9. https://doi.org/10.1542/peds.2014-3143.
246. Matricciani L, Olds T, Petkov J. In search of lost sleep: secular trends in the sleep time of school-aged children and adolescents. Sleep Med Rev. 2012;16:203–11. https://doi.org/10.1016/j.smrv.2011.03.005.
247. Belsky J, Pluess M. Beyond diathesis stress: differential susceptibility to environmental influences. Psychol Bull. 2009;135:885–908. https://doi.org/10.1037/a0017376.
248. Pluess M, Assary E, Lionetti F, et al. Environmental sensitivity in children: development of the highly sensitive child scale and identification of sensitivity groups. Dev Psychol. 2018;54:51–70. https://doi.org/10.1037/dev0000406.
249. Pluess M, Belsky J. Vantage sensitivity: individual differences in response to positive experiences. Psychol Bull. 2013;139:901–16. https://doi.org/10.1037/a0030196.
250. Pluess M. Individual differences in environmental sensitivity. Child Dev Perspect. 2015;9:138–43. https://doi.org/10.1111/cdep.12120.
251. Plass A, Wiegand-Grefe S. Kinder psychisch kranker Eltern: Entwicklungsrisiken erkennen und behandeln. Weinheim: Beltz; 2012.
252. Lawrence PJ, Murayama K, Creswell C. Systematic review and meta-analysis: anxiety and depressive disorders in offspring of parents with anxiety disorders. J Am Acad Child Adolesc Psychiatry. 2019;58:46–60. https://doi.org/10.1016/j.jaac.2018.07.898.
253. Wesseldijk LW, Dieleman GC, van Steensel FJA, et al. Do parental psychiatric symptoms predict outcome in children with psychiatric disorders? A Naturalistic Clinical Study. J Am Acad Child Adolesc Psychiatry. 2018;57:669–677.e6. https://doi.org/10.1016/j.jaac.2018.05.017.
254. Flouri E, Sarmadi Z, Francesconi M. Paternal psychological distress and child problem behavior from early childhood to middle adolescence. J Am Acad Child Adolesc Psychiatry. 2019;58:453–8. https://doi.org/10.1016/j.jaac.2018.06.041.

255. Witt A, Glaesmer H, Jud A, et al. Trends in child maltreatment in Germany: comparison of two representative population-based studies. Child Adolesc Psychiatry Ment Health. 2018;12:24. https://doi.org/10.1186/s13034-018-0232-5.
256. Schulte-Markwort M. Burnout-Kids: Wie das Prinzip Leistung unsere Kinder überfordert. München: Pattloch; 2015.
257. Eurostat. EU—Jugendarbeitslosenquoten in den Mitgliedsstaaten 2014. Hamburg: Statista; 2015. http://de.statista.com/statistik/daten/studie/74795/umfrage/jugendarbeitslosigkeit-in-europa/. Accessed 14 Jul 2015.
258. Collishaw S, Furzer E, Thapar AK, Sellers R. Brief report: a comparison of child mental health inequalities in three UK population cohorts. Eur Child Adolesc Psychiatry. 2019;28:1547–9. https://doi.org/10.1007/s00787-019-01305-9.
259. Resch F, Westhoff K. Adoleszenz und Postmoderne. In: Resch F, Schulte-Markwort M, editors. Kursbuch für integrative Kinder- und Jugendpsychotherapie. Weinheim: Beltz; 2008b. p. 67–76.
260. Lyotard JF. Beantwortung der Frage: Was ist postmodern? In: Engelmann P, editor. Postmoderne und Dekonstruktion: Texte französischer Philosophen der Gegenwart. Stuttgart: Reclam; 1990. p. 33–48.
261. Resch F. Psychotherapie und Realität. Z Kinder Jugendpsychiatr Psychother. 2015;43:81–3. https://doi.org/10.1024/1422-4917/a000336.
262. Ferraris M. Manifest des neuen Realismus. Frankfurt: Vittorio Klostermann; 2014.
263. Han B-C. Psychopolitik: Neoliberalismus und die neuen Machttechniken. 5th ed. Frankfurt: Fischer; 2014.
264. Huntington SP. Kampf der Kulturen: Die Neugestaltung der Weltpolitik im 21. Jahrhundert. München: Goldmann; 2002.
265. Rauschenbach T. Jugend—eine vernachlässigte Altersphase. DIJ Impulse. 2017;115:4–7.
266. Dornes M. Modernisierung der Seele: Kind—Familie—Gesellschaft. Frankfurt: Fischer; 2012.
267. Bauman Z. Flüchtige Zeiten: Leben in der Ungewissheit. Hamburg: Hamburger Edition; 2008.
268. Han B-C. Müdigkeitsgesellschaft. Berlin: Matthes & Seitz; 2010.
269. Ehrenberg A. Das erschöpfte Selbst: depression und Gesellschaft in der Gegenwart. Frankfurt: Campus Verlag; 2004.
270. Han B-C. Transparenzgesellschaft. Berlin: Matthes & Seitz; 2012.
271. Kashdan TB, Rottenberg J. Psychological flexibility as a fundamental aspect of health. Clin Psychol Rev. 2010;30:865–78.
272. Rosa H. Resonanz: eine Soziologie der Weltbeziehung. Berlin: Suhrkamp; 2016.
273. Orange DM, Atwood GE, Stolorow RD. Intersubjektivität in der Psychoanalyse: Kontextualismus in der psychoanalytischen Praxis. 1st ed. Frankfurt: Brandes & Apsel; 2015.
274. Stolorow RD, Brandchaft B, Atwood GE. Psychoanalytische Behandlung: Ein intersubjektiver Ansatz. Frankfurt: Fischer; 1996.
275. Resch F. Die psychische Struktur des Menschen und die Rolle der Musik. In: Schmidt HU, Stegemann T, Spitzer C, editors. Musiktherapie bei psychischen und psychosomatischen Störungen. München: Elsevier; 2019. p. 9–16.

Index

Printed in the United States
by Baker & Taylor Publisher Services